# Sensible Application of the ECG: A Pocket Guide

Kathryn Monica Lewis, RN, BSN, PhD
Phoenix, Arizona

Kathleen A. Handal, MD, DABEM
Scottsdale, Arizona

**DELMAR**

**THOMSON LEARNING**  Australia • Canada • Mexico • Singapore • Spain • United Kingdom • United States

## NOTICE TO THE READER

**Delmar Staff:**

| | |
|---|---|
| Director, Health Care Publishing: | William Brottmiller |
| Executive Editor: | Cathy L. Esperti |
| Executive Marketing Manager: | Dawn F. Gerrain |
| Acquisitions Editor: | Doris Smith |
| Developmental Editor: | Darcy M. Scelsi |
| Production Coordinator: | John Mickelbank |
| Production Editor: | Mary C. Liburdi |
| Project Editor: | Stacey Prus |

COPYRIGHT © 2001 Delmar, a division of Thomson Learning.
The Thomson Learning logo is a registered trademark used herein under license.

Printed in Canada

2 3 4 5 6 7 8 9 10 XXX 05 04 03 02 01

For more information, contact Delmar, 3 Columbia Circle, PO Box 15015, Albany, NY 12212-0515; or find us on the World Wide Web at http://www.delmar.com

Library of Congress Cataloging-in-Publication Data
Lewis, Kathryn Monica
    Sensible Application of the ECG: A Pocket Guide / Kathryn Lewis, Kathleen Handal
    p. ; cm.
    Includes bibliographical references and index.
    ISBN 0-7668-0522-0
    1. Electrocardiography—Handbooks, manuals, etc.   I. Handal,
Kathleen A.  II. Title.  [DNLM: 1. Electrocardiography—methods—
Handbooks. WG 39 L674 2000]
RC683.5.E5 L448 2000
616.1'297547—dc21                                          99-089617

*To Ed*

*To my mother, Evelyn Virginia Handal*

# Contents
....................................................................

**Chapter 6**
Junctional Rhythm and Junctional Arrhythmias 73

**Chapter 8**
Ventricular Ectopy, Ventricular Arrhythmias, Asystole, and
Pulseless Electrical Activity

# Foreword

······························································

A basic understanding of the mechanisms of cardiac arrhythmias and of their electrocardiographic presentation is one of
the most intellectually rewarding areas of patient care. At the
same time it constitutes the basis for correct decision-making
in choosing appropriate pharmacologic or electrical interventions if and when needed. Such therapy can culminate in a
hemodynamically-stable patient who moments before was in
an arrhythmia-induced crisis, or it may relieve symptoms cre-
ated by the arrhythmia in a stable patient. In either case correct
judgment is often predicated on an understanding of the
mechanism and the electrocardiographic diagnostic characteristics of the arrhythmia.

Dr. Kathryn M. Lewis, with Dr. Kathleen Handal, provides
in this text the kind of information that will enable readers to
advance their understanding of both the mechanisms of
arrhythmias and how they can be diagnosed on the electrocardiogram (ECG). In addition, they review the spectrum of therapy that may be needed to manage patients who need
intervention to achieve hemodynamic stability or relief of
symptoms. This book is really a sequel to the recently-pub-
lished books, *Sensible ECG Analysis* and *Sensible Analysis of the
12-Lead ECG*, itself a veritable treasure of facts presented in a
style that makes complex information easily understood, even
by the novice.

In many ways the *Sensible Application of the ECG: A Pocket
Guide* picks up where the previous texts left off. Here, the additional information gained from 12-lead electrocardiography is
presented, as well as diagnostic clues from single monitor leads.
The ECG manifestations of acute myocardial ischemia and
infarction are described and illustrated with singular clarity. At
the same time, we are reminded that the 12-lead ECG can be
very helpful in the differential diagnosis of tachyarrhythmias.
This is an area that is not fully appreciated, yet knowing what

clues to look for on the 12-lead ECG often can establish the specific diagnosis of wide-complex tachycardia and thus lead to the selection of the appropriate therapy. One example is an understanding of AV dissociation and how it can be identified in some ventricular tachycardia, as well as the QRS morphology in the 12-lead ECG when the tachycardia is ventricular in origin. Knowing what to look for on the ECG can reward both patient and provider of care when therapy is indicated.

When I read *Sensible ECG Analysis* I decided it should be recommended reading for all who wish to advance their understanding of cardiac arrhythmias. Now the *Sensible Application of the ECG: A Pocket Guide* takes my recommendation a step further. Like its predecessors, this book is a veritable storehouse of the kind of information that will make learning more about the mechanisms and ECG manifestations of arrhythmias a rewarding encounter.

Roger D. White
Professor of Anesthesiology
Mayo Medical School
Co-Medical Director
Gold Cross Ambulance Service
Rochester, MN

# Preface

......................................................

The ECG is established as an accurate tool for identifying arrhythmias. The ECG provides information about the source of the arrhythmia, the location of myocardial ischemia, injury, and infarction. This book provides essential information for the rapid recognition of arrhythmias and abnormal findings by using the surface and 12-lead ECG.

The format for this text is consistent and uniform, intended for quick reference. The text assesses and explains each ECG tracing and 12-lead ECG, listing characteristics, possible pathophysiology, probable mechanism, causes, and clinical implications. Proposed interventions are listed and examples presented. A list of abbreviations is provided, and a general reference for some medications is included.

The methods involved in patient assessment and management are developed as generic guidelines. In many instances the process is repetitive, to remind us to focus on the patient and not just the ECG. We presume that baseline assessment of the ABCs and assessment of pulses and circulation are generic to most clinical environments; therefore, they are not repeated for every arrhythmia discussed in the text. The same holds true for reassessment of the patient, vital signs, and the ECG in response to a chosen intervention.

## TO THE READER

We have exerted a great deal of diligence and effort to ensure that medications and dosages set forth in this text are in accord with current recommendations and practice at the time of this printing. In view of ongoing research and development in the laboratory and in clinical settings, and the continual influx of knowledge needed to apply any proposed intervention technique or to administer any medication. The clinician who is armed with knowledge of the patient's ECG and its clinical implications must have a strong, personal knowledge base before attempting patient care of any kind.

This book provides one basis of insight into a tool used to care for the patient in cardiac crisis. Although appearing to be prescriptive in approach and assessment, the book is not all-inclusive or futuristic in predicting new, improved medications and procedures. It is the provider's responsibility to maintain commitment to constant study and vigilance in order to provide optimal patient care.

Accurate interpretation of ECG tracings is vital in patient care. It is an available tool and, if used correctly, will help the clinician choose therapeutic modalities and interventions.

# Chapter 1
# Assessment and Management
# of the Cardiac Patient
••••••••••••••••••••••••••••••••••••••••••••••••••••••••••••

Each year in the United States, 1 million patients are admitted for unstable angina (USA) and almost the same number for myocardial infarction (MI). Rapid recognition and therapy given in the first few hours can significantly reduce mortality and evolution of the cardiac disease process. Clinical differentiation of acute MI and USA relies heavily on the presence or absence of electrocardiogram (ECG) findings. This tool is only of value if used and interpreted in the context of the patient's history and physical examination with detailed assessment of the cardiovascular system.

## PATIENT PRESENTATION

National statistics show that 5% of all acute myocardial infarctions (AMI) are actually misdiagnosed on initial presentation. The chief complaint of chest pain should be considered cardiac in origin until proven otherwise.

To the medical practitioner, "chest pain" refers to those terms commonly used by the patient to describe a discomfort, heaviness, tightness, or squeezing about one's chest or in one's chest. Chest pain due to cardiac disease can occur in almost all age groups.

It is important to remember that as many women as men suffer AMI. Women's symptoms often are less dramatic than men's, and there is a belief that women are less prone to AMI. Potential misconceptions such as this may delay the appropriate aggressive interventions.

It is important to be aware that patients' vocabularies differ. Patients' backgrounds, socioeconomic factors, and responses to pain and to their own bodies' sensations vary. Language barriers exist and are most dangerous when a false impression of understanding is assumed when little English is spoken. We are all individuals and express ourselves in a unique manner. Gender and age biases exist both in the home and workplace, and the clinician should not fall prey to this human failing.

The classic or textbook presentation of crushing, squeezing pressure in midchest or substernal that radiates to the neck and left shoulder and arm is not seen in the majority of cases. This classic scenario is least common in women and the elderly. Tolerance and affect play a role in the patient's manner and presentation during an acute MI.

Other chief complaints suggestive of cardiac disease are *syncope*, *dyspnea*, *palpitations*, dizziness, altered mental status, malaise, and hypotension. *New-onset atrial fibrillation* may be the only clue in some cases. Diabetics are notorious for presenting atypically when having a cardiac event. New-onset congestive heart failure and pulmonary edema as presentations are more common in the elderly. Relevant to all of these possible presentations is determining nature, onset, duration, intensity, previous similar episodes, associated symptoms, and frequency.

## PATIENT HISTORY

History taking is an art, because people are different not only in their bodies but how they experience and express sensations. Greeting the patient, maintaining eye contact, and touching while respecting personal space are part of the art. Understanding, patience, and word choice can help set a cooperative atmosphere. Being sensitive to the patient's comfort and feelings can enhance communication. Documentation, although important, should not intrude upon the patient-caregiver relationship. Lack of eye contact for a period with continued verbal questioning may be interpreted as impersonal care.

Listening to family members, companions, and caregivers allows the family unit to participate. This is important when there is a language barrier or when ethnicity or social mores indicate deference to a family member. Everything should be done to preserve the patient's integrity. Remember that the patient is suffering, so simple, short questions are best. Do not use a loud, arrogant, or impatient tone. Although there may be a need to be assertive in a confusing situation, most scenarios do not call for aggressively exerting control.

## CHIEF COMPLAINT

The chief complaint and symptoms associated with cardiac disease most commonly include chest pain/discomfort. Often a severe degree of pain is termed "sharp." The clinician will interpret this as the quality or character of the pain, whereas the patient equates "sharp" with intensity. Some say the pain feels like heartburn. This is a self-interpreted perception, and the clinician should ask when the sensation occurred prior to this encounter, and if and how it was resolved. It may help to encourage the patient to describe or relate the symptoms to previous experiences. To ensure proper interpretation, acknowledge your understanding of the answer. Volunteering terms and phrases with an explanation also may assist but should not be done prematurely lest the phrases lead the patient. This occurs when the clinician feels a sense of urgency and may be impatient to continue with care. The sense of timing for interrupting the patient is an important, acquired skill.

## OPQRST

In asking about the chief complaint, keep in mind OPQRST:

O = Onset/origin

P = Pertinent past history: time of onset, provocation, exertional, or nonexertional

Q = Quality: this is the patient's narrative description, for example, sharp, tearing, pressure, heaviness

R = Region/radiation: for example, arms, neck, back

S  =  Severity: have the patient use a scale where 10 = *severe* and 1 = *almost totally gone*

T  =  Timing: for example, when, after what activity

It is important to determine the location, as well as radiation, of the pain. Does the pain travel anywhere or seem to come from or go to another area? Pain may go to the jaw, to the neck, to one or both shoulders, and down one or both arms. Discomfort may also occur in the back, either straight through from the front or in a constricting band. Thoracic aortic dissection often is described as a tearing pain felt in the middle of the back.

Determining the duration or whether the pain is worsening or improving, is continuous or intermittent, or occurs at rest or with activity is an important factor in assessment of the cardiac patient. The reported duration of the pain may not be reliable. Asking focused questions to find out the exact time may be critical in deciding which therapy to initiate. Ask whether onset occurred relative to a meal, a TV show, a friend's visit or telephone call. These associations may increase the accuracy of the time of onset.

Important in the concept of duration is the degree of discomfort or intensity: Is it the worst angina you have ever had? Has the pain stayed constant or increased and tapered off? On a score of 1 to 10, what is it now? Many patients, when asked, "Do you have chest pain?" will answer, "No, it is a tightness; it feels like a weight is on my chest; it makes me feel like I can't breathe." Women may say, "My bra suddenly feels so tight." Relating the initial pain and intensity number enables communication with the patient and more accurately gauges treatment response.

Angina may be relieved by rest, without medication, and it may "just go away." This type may last less than 15 minutes. However, persistent, intense symptoms that last more than 15 minutes are of concern. Any chest discomfort, no matter the duration and especially if associated with other symptoms, is an emergency.

Precipitating factors or determining what the patient was doing when it started are also key information during an event.

Causes of onset may vary from emotional stress to physical exertion. Sudden temperature change or pain at rest or awakening from sleep carry a graver prognosis.

Aggravating or alleviating factors are helpful in developing the differential diagnosis. Actions such as moving one's arms or bending over that precipitate the pain can be meaningful. These pains are frequently described as sharp, knifelike, or stabbing. Pain brought on by breathing may be related to a musculoskeletal or pleuritic, lung-related problem. Only if the patient is stable, which is determined after a physical exam, should you ask the patient to perform the action that brings on or aggravates the pain. Knowing the factors that alleviate pain is important as well. For example, some mild hiatal hernia problems seem to improve when the patient is sitting upright. Belching or burping may improve chest pain if the pain has a gastrointestinal cause. However, patients with acute cardiac problems may also have gastrointestinal symptoms, especially if the inferior portion of the heart is involved. All of these symptoms may occur with myocardial ischemia, injury, and infarction.

Associated symptoms include belching, nausea, emesis (vomiting), diaphoresis, sweating, and cold or clammy skin. Vagal stimulation resulting from the MI can cause emesis and marked diaphoresis. *Dyspnea*, a sensation of inability to catch one's breath or inability to take a deep breath, is seen as a rapid almost gasping shallow breathing accompanying the pain. Palpitations without chest pain may be a presenting symptom of cardiac disease and may also be an associated sensation with cardiac pain. Palpitations are often described as a fluttering sensation, irregular beating, skipping, or "my heart is beating in my neck." No matter the nature or origin of the ectopy, the associated or primary symptoms of palpitations are concerning.

Significant history of the present illness includes determining if there have been any previous episodes. If so, what are the similarities and dissimilarities? Timing and frequency also can be helpful. Recent trauma or exertion out of the ordinary may be the etiology of the chest pain. Repetitive movements such as using the upper body can, over time, precipitate chest wall discomfort.

Questioning about past medical and medication history provides additional information, such as other illnesses, allergies, and surgeries. Asking about previous medical problems, specifically occurrence of congestive heart failure, heart attack, angina, hypertension, or chronic lung disease, is important.

For example, hypercholesterolemia is a significant risk factor. Because of vascular changes caused by the disease, diabetics (male and female) may voice very minor complaints, if any, when experiencing a cardiac event. They may not perceive, feel, or describe chest pain in the classic sense. Associated symptoms and signs may be the only clues. Knowing that the patient is a diabetic is also important. Recall, diabetes is an important risk factor for cardiac disease.

Find out if the patient has allergies; this may provide indirect information about not-yet-revealed medical conditions or problems.

Medication use, particularly nitrates (NTG, Isordil), beta-blockers, digitalis, diuretics, antihypertensives, antidysrhythmics, and calcium channel blockers, should be of particular interest to the clinician. Patients may not know the true category of their medications. Ask why the patient is taking a medication. For example, ask simple, straightforward questions such as, "Are you taking this for your blood pressure?" "Are you taking this for water retention?" Examples of medications that may flag a concern for the clinicians are nitrates (NTG, Isordil), beta-blockers (propranolol, atenolol), digitalis (Digoxin, Lanoxin), diuretics (Lasix, Maxzide, Dyazide), and antihypertensives (Vasotec, Prinivil). Antiarrythmics are of great importance and include Mexitil, Quinaglute, and calcium channel blockers (Calan, Procardia). Ask about regularity of use in a nonthreatening manner, because additions or omissions may precipitate a cardiac event. Changes of doses and recent stopping of medication are also relevant. Again, ask in a nonthreatening and nonjudgmental manner that will receive an honest response.

Another area of concern involves asking if the patient recently saw a physician and received medication in the office or was recently discharged from the hospital and was given unfamiliar medications. Sometimes cardiac medications have a long-lasting effect that may alter ECG measurements, for instance, amiodarone and tricyclic antidepressants prolong the QT interval. Asking the patient, "Did you or your doctor recently stop or change the dosage of a medication?" may provide essential clues to the immediate problem.

Some patients may deny heart problems, because they do not perceive a relationship between high blood pressure and heart disease. Use of cholesterol-lowering drugs may be the only clue that the patient has high cholesterol. Too often, patients feel that if they are on medication, they no longer have the disease or problem. The use of oral contraceptives or replacement hormone therapy often is not reported by the patient as a medication.

In addition, over-the-counter medications may precipitate a cardiac event. Often patients do not see these as worthy of mentioning, so you need to ask. Herbal homeopathic preparations can be cardiotoxic, for example, St. John's wort. Borrowing medications from family members or friends with "similar" problems is very common. In addition, recreational drugs such as cocaine can be cardiotoxic. Use of recreational drugs even in the relatively distant past can be a risk factor. To a recovering addict, 3 months of being "clean" is a "long time" of being drug-free. Therapy for concurrent illness and knowledge of the specifics of medication are important. Not only can this knowledge contribute to the diagnosis but it may help determine the type of intervention. Certain medications or recent procedures may negate the use of thrombolytics in the patient.

Social history gives clues to risk factors for cardiac disease. Recognized risk factors include smoking, diet including carbohydrate intolerance, sedentary living, obesity, personality type, and active psychosocial tensions. Alcohol abuse is another contributory factor to cardiomyopathy.

Family history for stroke, heart disease, diabetes, and hypertension; age of parents and siblings at death; known cholesterol levels; and vascular diseases all contribute to the patient history and can affect how quickly diagnosis can be reached.

## DETAILED PHYSICAL EXAMINATION

Examination of the patient, that is, the laying-on of eyes and hands, can be done rapidly and effectively to gather needed pairing of history with the state of the body. Explaining what you are going to do before touching the patient, especially when removing clothing, will ensure a quick physical examination. Explaining what you are going to do with various equipment is also important, because we tend to take for granted that everyone knows our tools. It is also important to let the patient know it will not hurt. Apprehension is usually easy to see; addressing a patient's fears will help eliminate any negative effect.

The physical examination as always begins with the initial assessment, addressing the life-threatening problems. The ongoing physical assessment begins while observing the total patient. Start with looking for dyspnea and tripod positioning, while observing the patient's expression. Is the patient fearful, agitated, angry, or frustrated? Are the eyes clear, bright, dull, or unseeing? Note the skin color, temperature, and hydration; jugular venous distention; and peripheral edema.

Additional clues are surgical scars, especially on the chest, that indicate previous heart surgery or the presence of a pacemaker. Often only the pacemaker prominence is seen on the chest. Look for a nitroglycerin patch on the chest, arms, inner thighs, or lower abdomen. Look for signs of obesity, questioning actual or estimated weight as necessary.

Listen to the major organs: the heart and lungs. Listen to breath sounds, assessing from base to apices and side-to-side. Sounds should be resonant, clear, and distinct. Report any adventitious sounds and, of course, absence of sound (pneumothorax—tension or surgical). Heart tones should be assessed at the apex and should be clear and distinct. Also important is auscultation for both carotid and abdominal bruits. Feeling or palpitating for equality of the pulses and for skin temperature and moisture can give clues to the state of the cardiovascular system. Listen as the patient speaks to you. Are the words clear and distinct, slurred, or muffled? Is the patient slow to respond?

Differentiating for the possible cause of chest pain/discomfort includes considering illnesses or insults that can occur in various organ systems. These include gastrointestinal, pulmonary, cardiac (including the great vessels) and the chest wall which includes ribs, muscles, and the costrochondral junction.

## THE PROCESS OF CARDIOVASCULAR ASSESSMENT

It is vital to know the patient's history and current status to determine whether the findings are appropriate for that patient. Then, changes in future assessments will indicate a deviation from normal. Observe general appearance, gross deformities, apparent nutritional status, posture, gait, cooperation, speech patterns, ability to speak in full sentences with or without difficulty, facial expression, and facial grimace during examination. Also note the reaction with family and friends when they are present, and when they respond to queries about the patient.

### Overall Inspection

**Skin:** Observe and record moisture, temperature, texture, turgor, thickness/thinness, edema, lesions, and changes in superficial vascularity.

**Nails:** Observe and record color, size, shape, and clubbing.

**Pulses:** Assess carotid, brachial, radial, popliteal, posterior tibial, and pedal. (Femoral is felt later, during palpation.) Assess for presence and equality.

*continues*

*continued*

**Neck:** Assess carotid pulses, as above. Assess jugular venous neck distention; ideally the patient should be positioned at a 45° angle.

**Chest:** Assess symmetry, precordial pulsations, and apical pulse for rate, rhythm, character, and intensity. Observe and record heaves, thrusts, thrills, vibrations, and pulsations.

**Abdomen:** Observe and record pulsations, edema, size, and symmetry. Assess the five *f*s of abdominal assessment: fluid, flatus, feces, fetus, and fatal tumor.

**Extremities:** Assess the skin and distal circulation. Note posterior of the legs for varicosities. Assess for tenderness, erythema, and Homan's sign. Assess fingers for nicotine stains.

## Auscultation

Auscultation is the examination performed with a bell/diaphragm stethoscope. High-frequency sounds are best heard with the diaphragm; low-frequency sounds are best heard with the bell of the stethoscope. Areas to auscultate include the neck, abdomen, and femoral areas for the presence of pulsation and bruits and equality of sounds.

### Auscultation of the Precordium

1. $S_1$ and $S_2$ are normal sounds.
2. $S_1$ is associated with ventricular systole and closure of the mitral valve.
3. $S_2$ is associated with ventricular diastole and closure of aortic and pulmonic valve.
4. Split $S_1$ and $S_2$ are abnormal systolic sounds.
5. $S_3$ and $S_4$ are abnormal diastolic sounds.
   - $S_3$ early diastolic sound associated with a dilated heart.

*continues*

*continued*

- $S_4$ caused by atrial contraction to a noncompliant ventricle. Often heard in the presence of acute MI. Cannot be distinguished with atrial flutter or fibrillation.
6. Gallops are abnormal diastolic sounds.
7. Snaps, staccato sounds that are sharp and higher in pitch than an abnormal diastolic $S_3$. Opening snap of the atrioventricular (AV) valve is heard before the second heart sound.
8. Clicks, systolic sounds that occur with valvular dysfunction. A click often occurs before a murmur.
9. Rubs, grating, high-pitched sounds heard throughout ventricular systole. Rubs are rarely heard over the same place twice. Rubs are affected by respiratory function and patient movement. Coughing can affect site of the rub.
10. Murmurs, vibrations that are heard over valves.
    - Systolic or ejection murmurs occur with valvular stenosis.
    - Diastolic murmurs occur over a valve that is insufficient.
11. Bruits, vibrations heard over stenotic vessels.
12. First-degree AV block with a reasonable heart rate may cause a muffled first heart tone.

## Palpation

### Cardiac Assessment by Palpation

Assess for presence or absence of rubs, thrills, or tenderness.
1. Anterior precordium over the xyphoid area (right ventricle).
   Apical area: Assess the point of maximum impulse (PMI). If there is an increase, this may indicate left

*continues*

*continued*

   ventricular hypertrophy (LVH). If shifted, this may
   indicate chronic obstructive pulmonary disease (COPD).
2. Pulmonic area: A thrill palpated here may indicate
   pulmonary stenosis, anemia, fever, or pregnancy.
3. Aortic area: A thrill palpated here may indicate aortic
   dilatation.
4. Epigastric area: Pulsations felt here may indicate
   aneurysm.

## Percussion

Use the flat of the fingers of the hand in contact with the part to
be palpated. Tapping is done with the third finger of the other
hand against the terminal joint of the third finger of the palpating
hand. Abnormal findings may occur when the examiner has
arthritis or a bony defect of the hand or fingers. Note that bone is
dense and air is not. Therefore, percussion over a solid surface (i.e.,
bone) is more dull than over air-filled surfaces such as the lungs.

### Terminology of Percussion

- Resonance: decreased density usually heard over lung
  tissue
- Impaired resonance: slightly more dense, may be
  caused by fluid filling otherwise aerated spaces
- Hyperresonance: lowest in density, heard over air-
  filled areas
- Dullness: a dense sound usually heard over dense tissue
- Tympany: very low density, over air-filled areas

## Vital Signs

Alterations of blood pressure, heart rate, core temperature, and
ventilatory status, to include pulse oximetry, are determining
factors in a cardiac event.

The carotid and radial pulses are palpated to determine rate and perfusion. Irregular rhythms can affect perfusion, for example, atrial fibrillation and flutter as well as any ectopy. With an irregular rhythm, listen to the apical pulse while palpating the radial to determine the extent of any deficit. Absence of a palpable carotid pulse with an ectopic beat is not a differential tool between ventricular and ectopic beats.

Before palpating the carotid, inspect the neck for abnormal pulsations. Auscultate with the stethoscope to determine presence of a bruit. This murmur-like sound implies a vascular rather than a cardiac problem. Decreased pulsations may be caused by decreased stroke volume but also may be due to atherosclerotic narrowing or occlusion. A tortuous and kinked carotid artery produces a unilateral pulsating bulge. During palpation it is possible to detect a thrill.

A carotid bruit with or without a thrill in a middle-aged or older patient suggests, but does not prove, arterial narrowing. A murmur that is aortic in origin may radiate up the carotid and simulate a bruit.

### Blood Pressure

Remember the basics: A proper size blood pressure (BP) cuff is critical and should be placed 2 to 3 cm above the antecubital area.

### Pitfalls in Taking Blood Pressure Readings

False high readings
- Cuff is too short, too narrow, or too loose.
- Patient arm is elevated above the heart level.
- Anxiety and anger can cause a high blood pressure.

Rapid deflation
- Can underestimate systolic pressure reading.
- Can overestimate diastolic pressure reading.

*continues*

*continued*

With obesity
- Place the cuff on the forearm and listen over the radial artery.
- For leg pressures, use a wide, long cuff on the lower one third of the thigh. Center the bag over the posterior surface and wrap snugly. Listen for sounds over the popliteal area.

Causes of weak and/or soft BP sounds:
- Incorrect placement of the stethoscope.
- Incorrect placement of the stethoscope and poor perfusion, and arrhythmias.
- Venous engorgement from incomplete deflation and repeated inflation.

## SUMMARY

The organized assessment of the cardiac patient is critical in determining the pathways of care. Associated diseases and therapies may conflict with many therapeutic modalities available to the practitioner. We have provided the baseline tool for organized approach to patient presentation, detailed physical examination, and an approach to obtaining a focused history. This chapter is not meant to be all-inclusive in the techniques and approach to patient assessment. It is the responsibility of the clinical practitioner to maintain commitment to the current knowledge and techniques based on the patient care standards in a specific work environment.

# Chapter 2
# The Electrocardiogram

## THE ECG LEADS

The ECG traces the variation in voltage produced by the heart muscle during depolarization and repolarization. The standard ECG records depolarization and repolarization along designated paths called lead systems.

A *lead* or *lead system* is an electrical picture of a heart's surface. Each lead traces the electrical activity between two points called electrodes. Electrodes of opposite polarity make up a bipolar lead. One positive electrode and a reference point make up a unipolar lead. Six limb leads (three bipolar and three unipolar) and six precordial leads make up the standard 12-lead ECG.

### The Limb Leads

The limb leads, I, II, III, aVR, aVL, and aVF, provide information about superior, inferior, rightward, and leftward forces.

Table 2-1 shows the heart surface reflected by leads I, II, and III.

**Table 2-1** Limb Leads and the Reflected Surface of the Heart

| Lead | Surface Viewed |
|------|----------------|
| I | Left free wall |
| II | Inferior, apical |
| III | Right inferior |

Leads I, II, and III are typically represented by a triangle that shows the spatial orientation of these leads (Figure 2-1). If the electrodes are placed correctly and the leads recorded simultaneously, voltage of the wave form in lead II should equal the sum of the voltages in lead I and lead III. In other words, lead I + lead III = lead II. If the R wave in lead II is not equal to the sum of lead I and lead II, the leads are not placed appropriately.

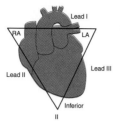

**Figure 2-1** Limb leads I, II, and III superimposed on the heart.

## The Augmented Leads

The two arm and the left leg electrodes are connected to a central reference point; the positive exploring electrodes can be paired with an indifferent reference point and are the unipolar leads aVR, aVL, and aVF (Figure 2-2). The *a* in aVR, aVL, and aVF stands for *augmented* or *amplified*, so named because these leads are automatically set to increase in size by 50% without any change in the configuration of the electrodes by the machine's property.

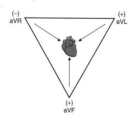

**Figure 2-2** The augmented leads in relationship to the heart.

## The Precordial Leads

The six precordial leads, also called the chest leads, are placed directly over the heart itself. They encircle the precordium and provide information about anterior, posterior, right, and left forces (see Table 2-2). The electrodes curve around the thorax over the heart (Figure 2-3), from the right ventricle, across the ventricular septum to the left lateral ventricular wall (Figure 2-4A). The right precordial leads are placed similarly on the right side of the chest (Figure 2-4B, Table 2-3).

**Table 2-2**  Placement of the Precordial Electrodes

| Lead | Placement |
| --- | --- |
| $V_1$ | Fourth intercostal space at the right sternal border |
| $V_2$ | Fourth intercostal space at the left sternal border |
| $V_3$ | Midway between $V_2$ and $V_4$ |
| $V_4$ | Fifth intercostal space at the midclavicular line |
| $V_5$ | Fifth intercostal space (same level as $V_4$) at the left anterior axillary line |
| $V_6$ | Fifth intercostal space (same level as $V_4$) at the left midaxillary line |

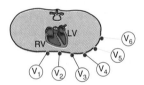

**Figure 2-3**  Precordial lead placement reflecting the heart.

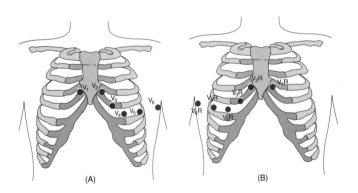

**Figure 2-4**  (A) Conventional precordial lead placement. (B) Right precordial lead placement.

**Table 2-3**  Placement of the Right Precordial Electrodes

| Lead | Placement |
|------|-----------|
| $V_{1R}$ | Fourth intercostal space at the left sternal border |
| $V_{2R}$ | Fourth intercostal space at the right sternal border |
| $V_{3R}$ | Midway between $V_{2R}$ and $V_{4R}$ |
| $V_{4R}$ | Fifth intercostal space at the right midclavicular line |
| $V_{5R}$ | Fifth intercostal space (same level as $V_{4R}$) at the right anterior axillary line |
| $V_{6R}$ | Fifth intercostal space (same level as $V_{4R}$) at the right midaxillary line |

The posterior surface of the left ventricle lies in a plane parallel to the frontal plane and is hidden from the precordial exploring electrodes by the anterior and septal surfaces. Infarctions of the posterior surface, usually by occlusion of the posterior descending coronary artery, may produce subtle electrocardiographic changes. Such damage will be reflected primarily in accentuation of depolarization forces over the anteroseptal surface in $V_1$ to $V_3$ as a mirror image of the posterior surface (Figure 2-5).

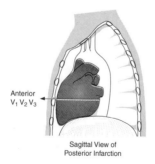

Anterior
$V_1$ $V_2$ $V_3$

Sagittal View of
Posterior Infarction

**Figure 2-5**  The position of the anterior precordial leads as they mirror the posterior surface of the heart.

## The MCL Leads

$MCL_1$ is a popular bipolar chest lead that simulates $V_1$ and is used to differentiate certain clinical conditions. In the 1960s,

Dr. Henry J. Marriott modified the bipolar chest lead, placing the positive electrode on the chest and the negative electrode on the left arm under the left clavicle. Thus, the modified chest lead in the $V_1$ position was termed $MCL_1$. Similarly, a positive electrode can be placed in the $V_6$ position for $MCL_6$.

The positions of the electrodes for $MCL_1$ and $MCL_6$ are illustrated in Figure 2-6, which shows the position of the electrode at the right sternal border between the fourth and fifth intercostal spaces, the same as in precordial lead $V_1$. The negative electrode does not change from the original placement; recall that it is indifferent in lead II, positive in lead I, and negative in $MCL_1$. Adjust the lead selector to lead I. $MCL_1$ may be helpful in visualizing some wave forms; however, it should not be used as the sole differential in some tachycardias.

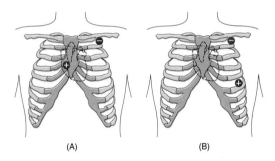

(A)                (B)

**Figure 2-6**  (A) In $MCL_1$, the negative electrode is under the left clavicle, and the positive is at the level of $V_1$. (B) In $MCL_6$, the negative electrode is under the left clavicle, and the exploring (positive) electrode is in the $V_6$ position.

## AXIS

The average direction of the spread of the depolarization wave through the ventricles as seen from the front is called the *cardiac axis* and is useful in deciding whether the flow of electrical depolarization is in a normal direction. The axis is derived from the QRS complex as seen in leads I, II, and III and sometimes, for simplicity, is called the net area of the QRS.

The axis is calculated for several reasons, some of which are to determine conduction defects within the bundle branch system and to help differentiate between ventricular ectopy and aberrant ventricular conduction.

Normal axis means that the depolarizing wave is spreading toward leads I, II, and III and, therefore, the net area of the QRS is seen as primarily positive. Because normal depolarization flows primarily inferior and to the left, the most positive wave form will be seen in lead II. So, if leads I and II are positive, no further calculation is necessary. If the QRS in lead I or lead II is negative, deviation in the mean flow of current exists.

Several methods are used to determine the extent or degree of deviation. There are degree assignments for each lead.

Lead I    = 0 degrees

Lead II   = +60 degrees (normal)

Lead III  = positive at +120 degrees (right), or negative at −60 degrees (left)

Lead aVF = positive at +90 degrees, negative at −90 degrees

Table 2-4 summarizes changes in polarity of the leads, identifying the need to calculate axis deviation.

**Table 2-4**  Changes in Limb Leads Indicating Axis Deviation

| Normal | Left | Extreme Left | Right |
|---|---|---|---|
| I(+) II (+) | I(+) aVF(−) | I(+) III(−) | I(−) II(+) |
| −30° to +110° | >−30° | >−60° | >+110° |

Assignment of degrees to the various leads is as shown with the help of the Lewis circle. Figure 2-7 illustrates the heart with the degree values assigned to the limb leads. Arrows are imposed on the circle to aid in calculation of the axis value. In Figure 2-7, lead I is positive so an arrow is drawn toward lead I. Lead III is the greatest negative, and an arrow is drawn away from the (+) of lead III. Lead aVL is also positive, but lead III has the greater value. Conclusion: Axis deviation is superior and to the left at −60°.

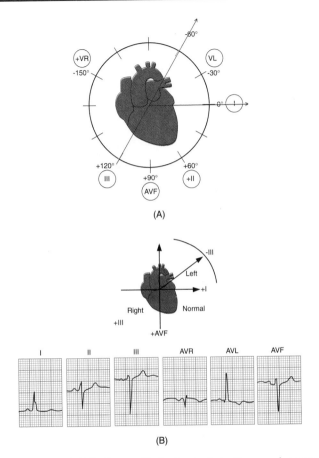

**Figure 2-7** (A) The heart with the Lewis circle. Degree values are assigned to the various leads, and arrows match the direction of the QRS in ECG below. (B) ECG tracing showing leads I and III being different in polarity. Leads I and aVL are positive, and lead III has the greatest negative net area.

When a more precise calculation is necessary, the hexaxial reference system is used. This is an intersecting pattern of six limb leads (Figure 2-8). The hexaxial reference system is used to determine the axis of the heart in the frontal plane; in other words, this will reference the flow of current as it occurs within the heart's conduction system. This is important clinically, because deviation from normal can aid in a differential diagnosis of many cardiac conditions and pathology within the ventricular conduction system.

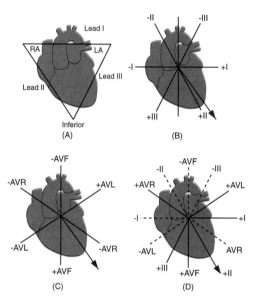

**Figure 2-8** Intersection of the lines of limb and augmented leads (A, B, C) as they form the skeleton of the hexaxial figure (D).

## Calculating Axis

The mean flow of current (axis) can be calculated in several ways. Since not all QRS complexes are clearly different in polarity or configuration, it is helpful to learn several methods. The most common and successful 2-step method is as follows:

1. Identify the equiphasic QRS.
2. Identify the lead that is perpendicular (at a right angle) and positive to this lead. (Remember, lead I is at a right angle to aVF, lead II is at a right angle to aVL, and lead

III is at a right angle to aVR. The flow of current, or axis, will be parallel to that lead.)

Figure 2-9 demonstrates the 2-step method of calculating axis.

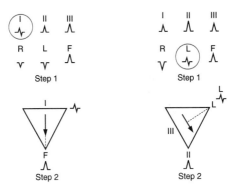

**Figure 2-9** Two examples of the 2-step method of calculating axis.

Another method is the quadrant method. This is successful when there are no equiphasic complexes or when there is more than one lead with equiphasic deflections.

1. Look at lead I and determine if the flow of current is to the right or the left; draw an arrow in that direction:
   a. A positive (+) QRS indicates the flow is to the left.
   b. A negative (−) QRS indicates the flow is to the right.
2. Look at lead aVF and determine if the flow is superior or inferior; draw an arrow in that direction:
   a. A positive (+) QRS indicates the flow is inferior, toward aVF.
   b. A negative (−) QRS indicates the flow is superior, away from aVF.
3. This creates a quadrant—look for the lead that is most positive in that quadrant. This will tell you the direction (axis) of current flow for that patient's QRS.

Figure 2-10 depicts an example of calculating axis using the quadrant method.

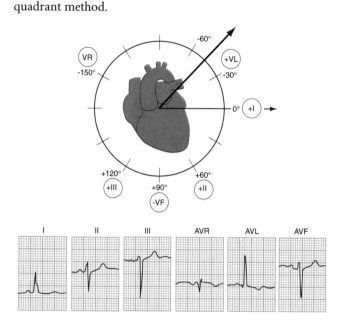

**Figure 2-10**  An example of calculating axis using the quadrant method. Lead I is positive, II is diphasic, and III is negative. Conclusion: left axis deviation at –60°.

Another quick method is the Handal–Lewis method:

1. Look at lead I—if the current flow is toward the right, lead I will be the most negative deflection.
2. Look at lead III—if the current flow is too far right (inferior), lead III will be very positive and the greatest positive deflection of all the limb leads. This is right axis deviation.

Summary of Causes for Axis Deviation:

Left Axis Deviation:

1. Left bundle branch block (LBBB)
2. Inferior wall myocardial infarction

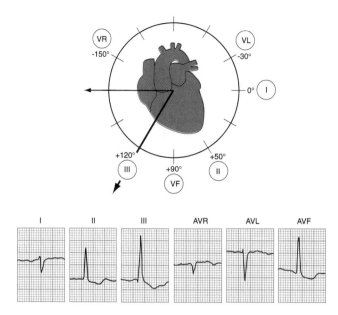

**Figure 2-11** An example of calculating axis using the Handal–Lewis method. Lead I is negative, and lead III is more positive than lead II. Conclusion: right axis deviation at (+)120°.

   3. Left anterior fascicular block
   4. Wolff Parkinson White syndrome
   5. Left ventricular hypertrophy—usually only with conduction delay

Right Axis Deviation:
1. Left posterior fascicular block
2. Right bundle branch block
3. Right ventricular strain (pulmonary embolism in an acute setting)
4. Wolff Parkinson White syndrome
5. Right ventricular hypertrophy—usually only with conduction delay

Figure 2-11 is an example of calculating axis using the Handal–Lewis method.

## CALCULATING HEART RATE AND RHYTHM

ECG monitors run at a standard rate and use paper with standard squares. Each small square is equal to 0.04 second. Each large square is made up of five small squares equal to 0.20 second. There are five large squares per second and 300 per minute. So, an ECG event such as a wave form representing ventricular activity, the QRS, that occurs once every large square is occurring at a rate of 300 per minute.

Amplitude, or voltage, is measured on the vertical, and each of the smallest blocks measures 0.1 millivolt (0.1 mV). The same small block measures height; each block measures 1 mm. Diagnostic ECG devices should be standardized so that l mV is equal to 10 mm. Figure 2-12 shows ECG monitoring paper and measurements.

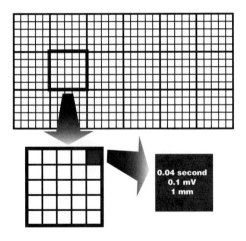

**Figure 2-12**  ECG monitoring paper and measurements.

Five small blocks on the horizontal would measure 0.20 second. Five blocks on the vertical would measure 5 mm and/or 0.5 mV. Note the darker lines that delineate five of the smallest blocks.

Estimating heart rate and evaluating duration and amplitude of wave forms are critical tasks in assessing the ECG. Time is measured on the ECG moving from left to right across the ECG paper. To calculate heart rate, use the ECG paper as a guide and, whenever possible, find a QRS that is on a heavy, vertical line. Count the number of large blocks between two consecutive QRS complexes, divide into 300, and thus calculate the estimated heart rate. With very rapid rhythms, count the number of very small blocks and divide into 1,500.

Remember this sequence: If the interval occurs every
 4 small squares, the rate is 375 per minute.
 5 small squares, the rate is 300 per minute.
 6 small squares, the rate is 250 per minute.
 7 small squares, the rate is 214 per minute.
 8 small squares, the rate is 188 per minute.
 9 small squares, the rate is 168 per minute.
 10 small squares, the rate is 150 per minute.

With slower rates, if the interval occurs every
 1 large square, the rate is 300 per minute.
 2 large squares, the rate is 150 per minute.
 3 large squares, the rate is 100 per minute.
 4 large squares, the rate is 75 per minute.
 5 large squares, the rate is 60 per minute.
 6 large squares, the rate is 50 per minute.

This method of calculation is shown in Figure 2-13 with ECG paper and an ECG rhythm. Counting the number of large squares (blocks) between QRS complexes (R-R interval) and dividing into 300 provides the estimated rate.

In the case of an irregular rhythm such as atrial flutter, atrial fibrillation, or sinus arrhythmia, the rate range should be calculated: first the widest (slower) of the R-R intervals, and then the narrowest (faster) of the R-R intervals. The calculated rate range is then reported. Figure 2-13 provides examples of regular and irregular rhythms and the estimated rates.

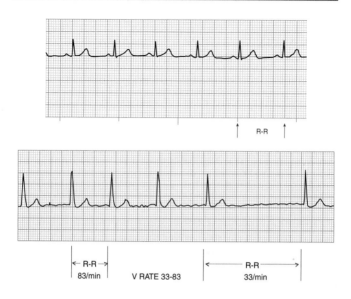

**Figure 2-13**  Calculating QRS rate with regular and irregular rhythms.

## WAVE FORMS

Several wave forms comprise the cardiac cycle. Figure 2-14 depicts the wave forms of the cardiac complex showing P, Q, R, S, T, and U waves and their measurements.

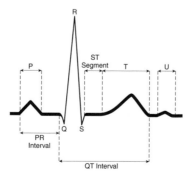

**Figure 2-14**  ECG wave forms and intervals.

## P Wave

Source: Represents synchronous atrial depolarization.

Duration: Less than 0.11 second.

Amplitude: Less than 3 mm.

Configuration: Symmetrical.

Polarity: Can be positive, negative, or diphasic depending on source and lead system.

Clinical significance of variations:

- Negative: When origin is from the AV junction or an atrial ectopic.
- Increased amplitude: May reflect enlarged atria or dilation secondary to mitral or tricuspid disease, hypertension, cor pulmonale, or congenital heart defect.
- Increased width and notching: May reflect right or left atrial enlargement (RAE or LAE). In RAE the initial notching is greater in amplitude, whereas in LAE the terminal notching is greater in amplitude.
- Diphasic: A wide negative component may reflect LAE.
- Peaked and notched: Taller in lead I than lead III may reflect right atrial enlargement.
- Absent: May reflect sinus block or arrest or a junctional origin.

## PR Interval

Source: Represents AV conduction time.

Duration: 0.12 to 0.20 second.

Clinical significance of variations:

- Less than 0.12 second with a normal QRS: May reflect Lown–Ganong–Levine syndrome.
- Less than 0.12 second with a wide QRS: May reflect Wolff Parkinson White syndrome.

- Greater than 0.20 second: May reflect AV conduction
  defect or the use of calcium-channel blockers or
  beta-blockers.

## QRS Complex

QRS is a relative term indicating ventricular depolarization
regardless of the wave forms that make up the complex (see
Figure 2-15).

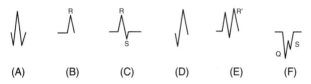

**Figure 2-15**   (A) QRS; (B) R; (C) Rs; (D) qR; (E) rSR′; (F) QS.

<u>Source:</u> Represents synchronous ventricular depolarization.

<u>Duration:</u> Less than 0.10 second.

<u>Amplitude:</u>

- Not less than 5 mm in II, III, aVF, $V_1$, and $V_6$.
- Not less than 7 mm in $V_2$ and $V_5$.
- Not less than 9 mm in $V_3$ and $V_4$.
- No more than 25 to 30 mm in any precordial lead.

<u>Causes of Low Voltage QRS:</u> Large chest AP diameter, poor
myocardial contractility, cardiomyopathy, previous MI with
loss of muscle mass, hypothyroidism, Addison's disease.
Also consider pericardial effusion due to infarction and
malignancy.

<u>Configuration:</u> Q is the first negative wave, R is the first pos-
itive wave, and S is next negative wave. A second R wave is
called R prime (R′). Similarly, a second S wave is called S
prime (S′).

<u>Polarity:</u>

- Narrow Q wave, 1 to 2 mm in I, aVL, and $V_6$.
- Narrow R wave, $V_1$ (may be absent).

Clinical significance of variations:

- Greater than 0.10 second: May reflect intraventricular conduction defect.
- Increased amplitude: May reflect ventricular hypertrophy or enlargement.
- Decreased amplitude: (Low voltage) may reflect pericardial effusion, emphysema, obesity, edema, diffuse coronary disease, or cardiac failure, large chest AP diameter, poor myocardial contractility, cardiomyopathy, previous MI with loss of muscle mass, hypothyroidism, or Addison's disease. Also consider pericardial effusion due to infarction and malignancy.
- Q waves: Presence may reflect necrosis. Must be judged within the clinical setting.
- Absent: May be affected by sinus block or arrest.

## ST Segment

Source: Represents early ventricular repolarization.

Polarity: Can be elevated 1 mm in leads I, II, and III, or 2 mm in precordial leads. Normally not depressed more than 0.5 mm in any lead unless reflecting early repolarization syndrome.

Clinical significance of variations:

- Elevated: Monophasic elevation greater than 1 mm above the line of the PR segment may reflect myocardial ischemia; concave elevation may reflect pericarditis; persistent elevation after resolution of MI may indicate ventricular aneurysm.
- Depression: Horizontal and depressed may reflect ischemia and subendocardial infarction. Negative, concave, curved (dig dip), and angular may reflect digitalis (see Figure 2-16C).

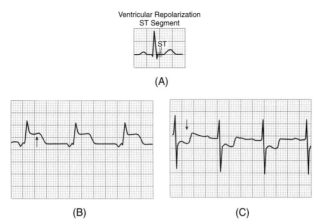

**Figure 2-16** (A) ST segment; (B) ST segment elevation; (C) ST segment depression.

## T Wave

Source: Represents synchronous ventricular repolarization.

Amplitude: No greater than 5 mm in standard leads and 10 mm in precordial leads.

Configuration: Asymmetrical, rounded.

Polarity:

- Positive in I, II, $V_3$, to $V_6$.
- Negative in aVR.
- Positive in aVL and aVF; may be negative if QRS is less than 5 mm.
- Varies in leads III, $V_1$, and $V_2$.

Clinical significance of variations:

- Negative: May indicate ischemia and infarction in lead facing the problem area.
- Notching: Rare except in children, may indicate non-conducted premature atrial complex (PAC); may indicate pericarditis.

- Increased amplitude: May indicate electrolyte imbalance or distortion because of a superimposed P′.
- Positive: Peaked with narrow base, symmetrical, and no measurable ST segment may reflect hyperkalemia. Opposite a premature QS that is a ventricular ectopic.
- Negative: Symmetrical, deep may reflect ischemia or infarction, cerebral ischemia, or hypokalemia. Opposite a premature QRS that is a ventricular ectopic. Post-extra systolic (–) T wave may occur because of transient ischemia produced by the ectopic beat (see Figure 2-17).

**Figure 2-17**  (A) T wave; (B) T wave inversion.

## QT Interval

<u>Source:</u> Represents total ventricular activity; depolarization (QRS) and repolarization (ST and T).

<u>Duration:</u> Less than one half the preceding R-R interval.

<u>Clinical significance of variations:</u>

- Prolonged: May be a normal variant or may reflect antiarrhythmic medications such as quinidine, procainamide, disopyramide, and amiodarone; may reflect hypokalemia, cerebral ischemia, hypothermia, or bradycardia (see Figure 2-18).

**Figure 2-18**  QT intervals.

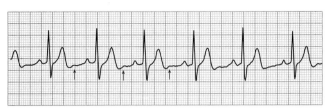

**Figure 2-19**  U waves.

**U wave**

  Source: Unknown.

  Amplitude: Low voltage.

  Polarity: Same as the T wave.

  Clinical significance of variations:

  - Increased amplitude: May reflect hypokalemia.
  - Reversed polarity: May reflect ischemia, left ventricular hypertrophy, or coronary artery disease (see Figure 2-19).

**SUMMARY**

The ECG wave forms represent electrical activity of the heart. Each wave form has a predictable appearance and measurement. Normal and consistent application of the principles for measurements will provide a sound foundation for ECG analysis.

# Chapter 3
# Complications and Management
# of the Cardiac Patient

••••••••••••••••••••••••••••••••••••••••••••••••••••••••••

## MANAGING THE PATIENT WITH CHEST PAIN

Management of the patient with chest pain includes the following:

1. Reassuring the patient.
2. Administration of high-flow oxygen.
3. Continuous monitoring to include 12 lead ECG.
4. Beginning an intravenous (IV) infusion of normal saline (NSS) or lactated Ringer's solution (LR; large-bore catheter).
5. Consider administering nitroglycerin (NTG) to patients with suspected cardiac pain, but whose blood pressure is reasonably stable.

While reassessing the patient, monitor the ECG rhythm and the medication effects, and note any ectopy that may be present. Anticipate hypotension and side effects such as lightheadedness, nausea, vomiting, or a sense of fright or feeling of impending doom expressed by the patient.

Administration of IV fluids may be enough to correct hypotension, should it occur. Reactions to NTG, along with possible pain relief, may include a transient flushing sensation and headache. Reassure the patient by explaining that the blood vessels are dilating, and the head is the most sensitive area, hence the head flush. Morphine sulfate also may be used to relieve pain; again, reassess the patient for relief, noting any side effects such as hypotension and decreased rate and depth of ventilation.

Ongoing care includes monitoring the patient for changes in blood pressure; heart rate, rhythm, and ectopy; and ST segment changes on the ECG.

Initial in-hospital evaluations may include 12-lead ECG analysis and may include right precordial ECG analysis and myocardial perfusion scanning. Serum lab analysis will be assessed for cardiac enzyme values. Medications may include the following:

1. Aspirin
2. Lidocaine, procainamide, magnesium, epinephrine, bretylium, amiodarone
3. Drugs that affect heart rate, such as atropine, adenosine, and verapamil
4. Calcium for problems related to the administration of calcium-channel blockers
5. Thrombolytic therapy to dissolve blood clots, such as tissue plasminogen activator (tPA) and streptokinase or urokinase, GPIIb/IIIa inhibition

Other treatments may include immediate balloon angioplasty, emergency bypass surgery, and insertion of the intra-aortic balloon pump (IABP). Insertion of a stent device may be considered to provide support and ensure patency of an intact lumen of a blood vessel.

## MANAGING THE CRITICAL COMPLICATIONS OF CARDIOVASCULAR DISEASE

Cardiac events, no matter what the insult, can result in grave conditions that require specific and immediate recognition and treatment. Among the possible sequelae are left ventricular failure, right ventricular failure, cardiogenic shock, and possibly cardiac arrest.

Other situations may arise, again depending on the basis of the insult to the cardiovascular system. These include the following:

1. Loss of vascular integrity, possibly secondary to rupture or occlusion of an arterial vessel. Depending on the caliber, arterial damage can be catastrophic.

2. Hypertensive emergencies.
3. Pulmonary artery occlusion from embolus can precipitate other life-threatening states.

Awareness of these potential complications is critical, because the sooner they are recognized, the more probable a favorable outcome.

## Cardiogenic Shock

Cardiogenic shock is the most severe form of pump failure. This occurs when the heart cannot meet the demands of the body and compensatory mechanisms are exhausted. Cardiogenic shock occurs after approximately 40% loss of left ventricle muscle wall function.

### *Clinical Implications*

1. Hypotension (systolic <80 mm Hg)
2. Altered level of consciousness
3. Sinus tachycardia
4. Cool and clammy skin
5. Pulmonary edema (usually present)

### *Management*

1. Assess and secure an airway.
2. Administer high-flow oxygen.
3. Position of comfort: The patient is usually in a supine position and an IV infusion begun.
4. Medications for cardiogenic shock, may include the following:
   a. Dopamine
   b. Norepinephrine
   c. If pulmonary edema is present
      - Morphine
      - Nitroglycerin
      - Furosemide
      - Oxygen with positive pressure ventilation (PPV).

## Cardiac Arrest

Cardiac arrest/sudden death, defined as death within an hour of onset of symptoms, accounts for 60% of all deaths from coronary artery disease.

### *Causes*

- Atherosclerotic heart disease
- Arrhythmias (V-fibrillation)
- Drowning
- Electrocution
- Electrolyte and acid-base imbalances
- Hypothermia
- Trauma
- Drug overdose
- Hypoxia
- Pulmonary embolism
- Stroke

### *Management*

1. Cardiopulmonary resuscitation (CPR).
2. Airway management to include intubation.
3. Defibrillation for pulseless ventricular tachycardia or fibrillation should be done without delay.
4. Transcutaneous or transvenous cardiac pacing may be effective for bradycardia and may be considered in asystole.

Management of arrest due to pulseless electrical activity (PEA) includes the following:

1. CPR
2. Intubation and ventilation
3. Identification of the cause
   a. Tension pneumothorax—assess bilateral breath sounds
   b. Hypovolemia—fluid challenge

   c. Severe electrolyte imbalance—lab analysis for hyper-kalemia and hypokalemia

   d. Hypoxia—high flow oxygenation, ventilation at 12 to 20 breaths/minute; assess pulse oximetry and/or end-tidal $CO_2$ values

   e. Infarction resulting in loss of wall motion—question pulses with CPR compressions

   f. Myocardial rupture—question pulses with CPR compressions

   g. Tamponade—question pulses with CPR compressions

   h. Severe acidemia—assess pH, $PACO_2$, and arterial oxygen tension

   i. Drug overdose—patient/bystander history

   j. Pulmonary embolus

## VASCULAR EMERGENCIES

Vascular emergencies include complications due to occlusion, dissection, infection, inflammation, trauma and congenital anomalies.

### Aneurysm

An aneurysm is a circumscribed dilation of an artery connection with the lumen of an artery. This condition in arteries is caused by ballooning of an arterial wall as a result of a defect or weakness in the wall layers. Most aneurysms that become noticed are in high-pressure vessels such as the aorta. Aortic aneurysm can occur in the arch of the heart or in the abdomen near the renal arterial branches.

The most common location is the abdominal aorta between the renal arteries and iliac bifurcation. Abdominal aortic aneurysm (AAA) most commonly results from atherosclerosis. This condition is more common in males, usually between 60 and 70 years of age.

### Signs and Symptoms

- Abdominal pain
- Back and flank pain that is often described as a "tear-ing sensation"
- Urge to defecate
- Pulsating mass
- Decreased femoral pulse
- History or presentation of gastrointestinal (GI) bleeding
- Hypotension that occurs with dissection

The patient with a history of hypertension may be normotensive before the event. No extensive palpation should be performed. Management is surgical repair as soon as possible.

## Aortic Dissection

Aortic dissection occurs after a small tear in the inner wall of the aorta. Blood enters and creates a false passage within the vessel wall.

### Causes

- Hypertension is the major predisposing factor.
- Prevalence in the 40 to 50 age group.
- Family history of cardiac and/or vascular problems.

### Signs and Symptoms

- Ripping or tearing substernal pain radiating to the back
- Hypertension
- Syncope
- Stroke
- Absent or reduced pulses
- Pain between the shoulder blades. The patient may report the pain changes location over time

*continues*

> *continued*
> - Heart failure
> - Pericardial tamponade
> - AMI

## *Management*

1. Rapid transport to definitive surgical care
2. Supporting the patient's ABCs with high-flow oxygen
3. IV normal saline (NS) or Ringer's lactate for volume expansion (RL)
4. Control and monitoring of blood pressure

### Traumatic Aortic Rupture

Traumatic aortic rupture (TAR) is caused by blunt or penetrating trauma. Prognosis is grave should the aorta rupture. TAR can be treated surgically if detected before complete rupture.

> ### *Causes*
> - Car crash with severe intrusion into the vehicle
> - Blunt trauma sustained when thrown from a vehicle
> - Blunt trauma when hit by an object such as a ball, bat, or large, heavy object dropped onto the victim's body
> - Fall injury

## *Management*

1. CPR if pulseless
2. Rapid transport to level I trauma center whenever possible
3. IV fluid infusions
4. May consider cessation of efforts depending on current clinical standards

## Acute Arterial Occlusion

Acute arterial occlusion is a sudden occlusion of arterial blood flow to an organ. The most common artery this occurs in is the mesenteric artery.

*Causes*

- Embolus
- Thrombus
- Trauma
- Tumor
- May be idiopathic

*Signs and Symptoms*

- Pain
- Pallor
- Paralysis
- Paresthesia
- Pulselessness

Early recognition before the bowel becomes infarcted can be life-saving. Acute management involves supporting vital signs until the condition can be resolved.

## Acute Pulmonary Embolism

Acute pulmonary embolism (PE) is a traveling blood clot or particle that lodges in a pulmonary artery. Sources are air emboli, fat emboli, amniotic fluid, and a blood clot.

*Causes*

- Immobilization
- Thrombophlebitis
- Medications
- Increased pulmonary vascular resistance
- Increased pulmonary pressure
- Ventilation/perfusion mismatch

*Signs and Symptoms*

Signs and symptoms will depend on the size of vessel that becomes occluded.

- Usually a sudden onset of severe, unexplained dyspnea occurs, usually with chest pain.
- Evidence of right heart failure with hypotension from decreased left ventricular filling.
- Recent history of immobilization or surgery.

Management of PE includes acutely supporting vital signs and swift use of anticoagulation therapy.

**HYPERTENSIVE EMERGENCIES**

A hypertensive emergency is an elevation of blood pressure (diastolic BP usually >130 mm Hg) that threatens function of the heart and brain.

**Signs and Symptoms**

- Altered mental status
- Restlessness
- Confusion
- Blurred vision
- Nausea and vomiting

Hypertensive encephalopathy may lead to congestive heart failure (CHF) or stroke.

**Management**

1. High-flow oxygen
2. IV infusion for administration of medications

Careful titration of blood pressure for precise control and monitoring can greatly reduce the mortality and morbidity of this dangerous condition.

## Peripheral Vascular Conditions

Noncritical peripheral vascular conditions include deep venous thrombosis and inflammation and thrombosis of a vein. Most commonly this occurs in the larger thigh and calf veins.

### Causes

- Aneurysm
- Atherosclerosis
- Immobilization
- Infection
- May be idiopathic
- Peripheral arterial atherosclerotic disease
- Permanent dilation and tortuosity
- Thrombosis
- Trauma
- Tumor

### Signs and Symptoms

- Pain, sudden or gradual onset
- Pallor
- Paralysis
- Paresthesia
- Pulselessness
- Swelling
- Tenderness
- Homan's sign (acute pain with dorsiflexion of the foot)
- Skin pale or mottled distal to or over the affected area
- Skin temperature may vary; may be warm and red, or may be cool, reflecting diminished circulation to the affected area or extremity

*continues*

*continued*

- Skin may be moist or dry, reflecting diminished circulation to the affected area or extremity
- Discomfort may radiate or remain localized
- Claudication (a condition caused by ischemia of the muscles, characterized by attacks of lameness or pain)
- Peripheral pulses absent or diminished over the affected extremity
- May note unequal blood pressure in each arm
- Bruit over affected vessel(s)

### Clinical Implications

1. Pulmonary embolus
2. Hemorrhage
3. Mesenteric occlusion
4. Stroke

### Management

Focus is on dissolving the thrombus while avoiding dislodging or tearing the thrombus and creating an embolism. Immediately elevate the legs to promote venous return.

## Varicose Veins

Varicose veins are caused by dilation of superficial veins.

### Causes

- Congenital dilation
- Tortuosity
- Incompetent valves
- Occupations requiring long periods of standing
- Pregnancy

*Signs and Symptoms*
- Visible distention over the vessel
- Swelling of the extremity over the affected area
- Discomfort
- Skin color changes

This is generally a nonthreatening condition, but varicose veins may rupture, causing brisk bleeding that can usually be controlled by direct pressure and elevation of the area.

## Peripheral Arterial Disease

Peripheral arterial disease is often associated with diabetes.

*Causes*

- Aneurysm
- Atherosclerosis
- Immobilization
- Infection
- May be idiopathic
- Permanent dilation and tortuosity
- Thrombosis
- Trauma
- Tumor

*Signs and Symptoms*
- Foot circulation problems
- Pretibial hair loss
- Red skin color in dependent extremities

Peripheral arterial disease may lead to gangrene and is not a medical emergency unless occlusion occurs.

## MANAGEMENT TECHNIQUES IN EMERGENCY CARDIAC CARE

Basic life support is a primary skill for managing pulseless patients, and the technique should be reviewed frequently. Critical assessment of the technique during CPR is crucial to the success of the procedure and prevention of complications. Assessment should include pneumothorax, myocardial contusion, chest wall contusion, and liver and splenic damage.

### Precordial Thump

Precordial thump is used to stimulate a depolarization within the heart and may allow resumption of natural rhythm. The thump is used to convert ventricular tachycardia (VT) and V-fib in witnessed situations when a defibrillator is unavailable. It is not recommended in pediatric patients.

Technique for delivery of the precordial thump is to use the heel of a fist to deliver a blow to the midsternum from a height of 10 to 12 inches. Deliver the thump along the long axis of the sternum to avoid rib damage.

### ECG Monitoring

Monitoring heart rate and rhythm using a monitor or monitor/defibrillator can include 2-lead, 3-lead, and 12-lead analysis. Using the quick-look technique through chest paddles is an option when electrodes malfunction and the patient is in cardiac arrest.

Causes of poor readings include excessive body hair, diaphoresis, loose or dislodged electrodes, dried conductive gel, inaccurate placement of electrodes, patient movement, muscle tremor (involuntary movement or spasm of a muscle or muscle group), broken patient cable or lead wire, low battery, and faulty grounding or a defective monitor.

### Defibrillation

Defibrillation is the definitive treatment for ventricular fibrillation; sustained, pulseless ventricular tachycardia; and torsade de pointes. Defibrillation delivers an electrical current that passes through a critical mass of myocardium to depolarize myocardial cells. It allows cells to repolarize uniformly so a more normal rhythm can be restored. It causes an intense vagal-like response.

Defibrillation generally uses a DC-powered electrical capacitor that delivers energy expressed in joules across a chest wall. Resistance to defibrillation includes chest wall density, tissue, muscle, bone, blood, and oils added to the skin. Position of the paddles, use of conductive media, and amount of energy decrease resistance to the defibrillating current. Research is continuing to evaluate whether indirect current defibrillation may be more effective.

Conversion is difficult in the presence of acidosis, hypoxia, hypothermia, electrolyte imbalance, and drug toxicity. Heart size and body weight are considerations for determining paddle size and placement. Paddle/skin interface is necessary to decrease skin resistance. Paddle contact pressure should be a firm, downward pressure.

## Synchronized Cardioversion

Synchronized cardioversion is the delivery of an electrical shock to the heart so it coincides with the R wave and thus, avoids the heart's relative refractory period. Indications for synchronized cardioversion are sustained paroxysmal supraventricular tachycardia (PSVT) and atrial fibrillation with rapid ventricular rate range. Atrial flutter, with ventricular rate at 150/minute, may also be considered for synchronized cardioversion. Energy requirements for synchronized cardioversion are sometimes based on the arrhythmia involved and physician direction.

Valsalva maneuvers and carotid sinus massage are used to convert PSVT by stimulating baroreceptors in carotid bodies; the increased vagal tone may decrease heart rate. Carotid massage should be used with caution, especially in the older adult. The carotid arteries should be auscultated by the physician, assessing for bruit. Absence of bruit does not rule out plaque, which is important because dislodgment of plaque may cause cerebral incidents such as stroke.

### SUMMARY

The choice of interventions in managing the patient with cardiac compromise is a wide topic. We have provided the baseline tool for an organized approach to patient care. This chapter is not meant to be all-inclusive in the techniques. It is the responsibility of the clinical practitioner to maintain a commitment to current knowledge and techniques based on the patient care standards in a specific work environment.

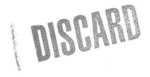

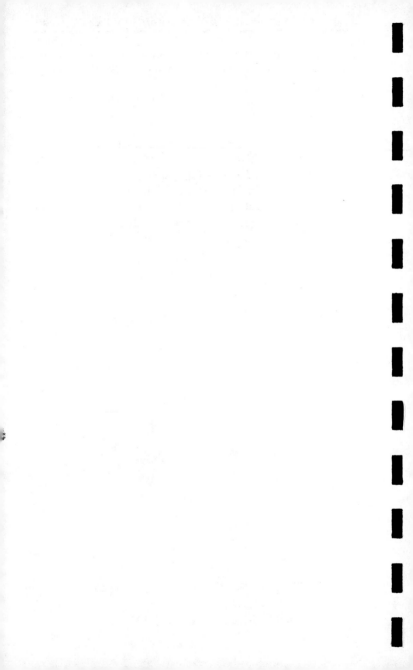

# Chapter 4
# Medications, Electrolytes, and the ECG
•••••••••••••••••••••••••••••••••••••••••••••••••••

Numerous medications and electrolyte imbalances can influence the heart's electrical function, altering the duration and amplitude of ECG wave forms. Similarly, ST segment elevation, depression, coving, and arrhythmias can be induced by medications.

Antiarrhythmic medications used for noncardiac conditions will alter the patient's ECG tracing. Examples of this include the use of beta-blockers for migraine therapy, timolol eye drops for control of glaucoma, and calcium-channel blockers for control of hypertension. To recognize all the possible causes for ECG changes, the clinician should carefully take a medical history. As with any other diagnostic tool, clinical correlation is imperative.

Treatment modalities dealing with the causative conditions and specific pathologies are beyond the scope of this text.

## MEDICATION-INDUCED CHANGES ON THE ECG

The unexpected effects on the heart by medications given for any reason warrant attention, as do the effects from medications given to treat cardiac problems. Interpretation and anticipation of possible outcomes and knowledge of the adverse effects of specific medications alone or in combination can be critical. Medications alone may produce visible ECG changes including increases in heart rate and prolonged PR intervals, as is the case with antidepressants.

Although many ECG changes are produced by antiarrhythmic medications, these changes may not be present in all ECG leads and may vary from individual to individual. Many medications are known to prolong the QT interval and, therefore, cause ventricular arrhythmias. Patients, even without underlying heart disease, who take medications that alone or in combination with another medication cause prolonged QT intervals can develop life-threatening arrhythmias.

Patients with already congenital QT intervals can develop ventricular arrhythmias as a result of taking medications that prolong the QT interval. Concomitant use of medications known to prolong the QT interval will increase the risk of an arrhythmia. Included in this category are certain of the following types of drugs:

1. Antiarrhythmics
2. Antipsychotics
3. Antidepressants
4. Anti-anginal drugs such as bepridil (Vascor®)
5. Antifungal medications taken orally or intravenously
6. Azole class (difflucon, fluconazole)
7. Broad-spectrum antimicrobials such as erythromycin, clarithromycin (Biaxin®) and sparfloxacin (Zagam®)
8. Calcium-channel blockers
9. Neuroleptic agents
10. Tricyclic antidepressants

The preceding list is not an exhaustive review of all possible medications that can effect the heart's normal conduction and functioning. We next address the medication effects most frequently reported and encountered in general medical practice.

### Digitalis

Digitalis preparations (Lanoxin™, Digoxin™) are used to treat patients with heart failure and certain arrhythmias. One of the effects of digitalis is to shorten ventricular repolarization. ECG changes reflecting digitalis effect does not imply toxicity. Digitalis toxicity is potentiated and the toxicity is considered "prorhythmic" in the settings of ischemia, low serum potassium and magnesium levels, high calcium levels, and hypothyroidism. Toxicity must be proven with lab analysis and clinical presentation.

## ECG Characteristics

- Shortening of the ST segment and T wave.
- Negative ST coving or scooping. This change is sometimes called the *dig effect* or termed *dig dip*.
- ST segment and T wave are often fused so that clear distinction between the two is impossible.
- Prominent U waves

## Digitalis-Induced Arrhythmias

- Atrial flutter with junctional escape rhythm
- Atrial tachycardia
- Atrial tachycardia with AV block
- Atrial fibrillation with junctional escape rhythm
- AV junctional tachycardia
- Bidirectional ventricular tachycardia (right bundle-branch-block [RBBB] and QRS alternans in $V_1$)
- Idiojunctional rhythm
- Premature ventricular complexes (PVCs)
- Sinus or AV Wenckebach phenomenon
- Sinus bradycardia (see Figure 4-1)

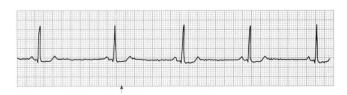

**Figure 4-1** Sinus bradycardia at 37/minute, ST segment depression (coving).

## Anti-Arrhythmic Agents

1. Type IA agents, Sotalol, (Betapace), increased QT interval
2. Type IC (flecainide (Tambocor), encainide, (Enkaid)) may cause sudden cardiac death in ischemic patients.
3. Quinidine may induce arrhythmias which may increase mortality

## Broad-Spectrum Antibiotics

Certain antibiotics, especially erythromycin, affect the QT interval. Included are clarithromycin (Biaxin®), a semisynthetic oral macrolide antibiotic. Although IV administration is more precarious, oral dosing can affect the ECG. A single standard dose of IV erythromycin prolongs the QT interval. Therefore, it is recommended that the drug always be administered as a slow infusion and the patient and the ECG carefully monitored.

This ECG effect may be reversible once the medication is discontinued. ECG monitoring especially in critically ill patients should accompany any course of IV erythromycin therapy. This precaution is warranted for patients with possible electrolyte disorders and for patients taking other drugs with similar cardiac effects (Mishra, Friedman, & Sinha, 1999).

Newly emerging synthetic broad-spectrum antimicrobials, for example, sparfloxacin (Zagam®), carry warnings regarding use with patients taking antiarrhythmic drugs and patients with a prolonged QT interval.

## Neuroleptic Drugs

A frequently used class of medication, Phenothiazine and Butyohenone tranquilizers can cause reversible Q and T wave distortion. Chlorpromazine (Thorazine™) especially at high doses causes QT interval prolongation. Again, careful history taking and correlation with the physical examination will place such ECG changes in the proper context (Warner, Barnes, & Henry, 1996).

## Tricyclic Antidepressants (TCA)

Prolonged QT and widened QRS intervals are seen in patients taking this class of medications. They are prone to precipitate arrhythmias especially in those persons with preexisting cardiac conditions. Prolonged QT intervals may progress to Torsade de Pointes or cardiac arrest.

These drugs are used with caution in the setting of arrhythmias and QTc prolongation. Aside from the sinus tachycardia due primarily to anticholinergic effects, TCA-toxic changes seen on the ECG are primarily attributed to the sodium channel blockage caused by these agents. The majority of patients at significant risk for developing cardiac or neurological toxicity will have a QRS complex greater than 0.10 second or a rightward shift of the terminal 40ms of the frontal plane QRS vector.

### ELECTROLYTE ABNORMALITIES

Electrolytes are present in a specific equilibrium, allowing for proper functioning of the body at the cellular level. Many biochemical diseases create an imbalance. Although signs, symptoms, and laboratory analysis will help monitor for any discrepancy, the ECG can also reveal electrolyte changes.

### Hyperkalemia

Hyperkalemia is a greater than normal concentration of potassium ions in the blood. Increased levels of serum potassium will decrease myocardial resting membrane potential. Potassium levels greater than 6.0 mEq/L may result in the following (see Figure 4-2):

1. Narrow, peaked, tented T waves
2. Prolonged PR intervals
3. Decreased P wave amplitude
4. Prolonged QRS complexes

As serum potassium levels increase, the QRS becomes distorted and takes on an undulating appearance.

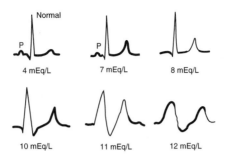

**Figure 4-2** Hyperkalemia.

### Common Causes

- Potassium supplement overdose
- Acidosis
- Anoxia
- Oliguria
- Renal failure
- Soft tissue trauma

## Hypokalemia

Hypokalemia, an abnormally low concentration of potassium ions in the blood, causes an increase in resting membrane potential. If hypokalemia persists, there is an increase in Phase 4 depolarization within the Purkinje fibers. This contributes to spontaneous ectopics. Fibers become nonexcitable as the resting potential becomes less and less negative. Finally, as huge U waves begin to appear, the patient is vulnerable to torsade de pointes.

Potassium levels less than 3 mEq/L cause the following (see Figure 4-3):

1. ST segment depression
2. U waves that may merge with T waves
3. Flattening of T waves

4. U waves that may also increase to a size greater than the amplitude of the T wave (serum levels <2 mEq/L)
5. Concurrent use of digitalis preparations leads to bradyarrhythmias and PVCs (see digitalis-induced arrhythmias).

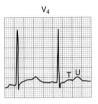

**Figure4-3**  Hypokalemia: serum potassium 2.2 mEq/L.

**Common Causes**

- Diuretic therapy without concurrent use of potassium
- Gastric suctioning
- Persistent diarrhea
- Prolonged bouts of emesis

## Hypercalcemia

Hypercalcemia occurs with calcium levels greater than 11mg/DL. Uncorrected hypercalcemia can result in seizure, coma, and death. The significant ECG change with hypercalcemia is a shortened QT interval (see Figure 4-4).

**Common Causes of Hypercalcemia**

- Adrenal insufficiency
- Breast and lung cancer
- Estrogens
- Idiopathic hypercalcemia

*continues*

*continued*

- Lithium
- Multiple myeloma
- Primary hyperparathyroidism
- Prolonged immobilization
- Renal failure
- Sarcoidosis
- Thyrotoxicosis
- Vitamin D intoxication
- Vitamin A intoxication

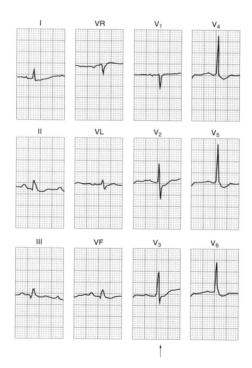

**Figure 4-4** Hypercalcemia.

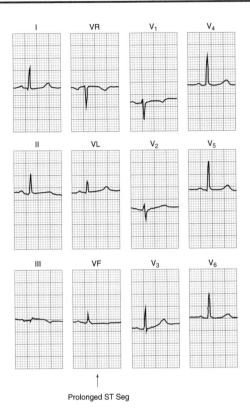

Prolonged ST Seg

**Figure 4-5** Hypocalcemia.

## Hypocalcemia

Hypocalcemia, defined as a serum calcium level less than 8 mg/DL, lengthens the refractory period. The significant ECG change with hypocalcemia is a lengthening of the QT interval (see Figure 4-5).

**Common Causes**

- Diuretics
- Hyperphosphatasemia
- Hyperventilation
- Hypomagnesemia secondary to release of parathyroid hormone
- Hypomalacia in adults
- Hypoparathyroidism
- Respiratory alkalosis
- Rickets in children
- Sepsis
- Small bowel bypass

Table 4-1 summarizes ECG changes induced by some medications and electrolyte imbalances. These changes must be correlated with clinical history and serum levels.

**Table 4-1** ECG Changes Resulting from Medication and Electrolyte Imbalances

| ECG Wave Forms/Complexes | Medication* | Electrolyte Imbalance |
| --- | --- | --- |
| P wave amplitude ↓ | | Hyperkalemia |
| P wave notched | Quinidine | |
| PR interval >0.20 second | Digitalis Procainamide Quinidine Verapamil | Hyperkalemia |
| QRS complex >0.10 second | Bretylium Disopyramide Lidocaine Procainamide Quinidine Tricyclic antidepressant | Hyperkalemia |

*continues*

**Table 4-1** *Continued*

| ECG Wave Forms/Complexes | Medication* | Electrolyte Imbalance |
|---|---|---|
| ST segment ↓ | Digitalis Quinidine | Hypokalemia |
| T wave amplitude ↓ | Digitalis Procainamide | Hypokalemia |
| T wave amplitude ↑ | Quinidine | Hyperkalemia |
| T wave ↓ | Digitalis Procainamide | Hypokalemia |
| U wave amplitude ↑ | | Hypokalemia Hypomagnesemia |
| QT interval ↓ | Bretylium Lidocaine | Hypercalcemia |
| QT interval ↑ (may also be a normal variant) | Neuroleptics GI stimulants Certain antibiotics Antiarrhythmics Antifungals Certain herbal supplements | Hypocalcemia |

* ECG measurements are sensitive to many drugs with antiarrhythmic potential, including medications taken for other reasons, for example, calcium-channel blockers for hypertension and beta-blockers for angina. This is not an all-inclusive list.

## SUMMARY

This chapter alerts the clinician to the ability of medications to alter ECG patterns. The chapter does not exhaustively list of all the possible proarrhythmia medications or list all other classes of medications that can affect the ECG.

The reader is urged to check package inserts for each drug suspected of altering the patient's electrolyte balance and the ECG. The continual flow of information relating to drug therapy and drug reactions, dosages, warnings, and precautions is particularly vital when the medication or supplement is new.

## REFERENCES

Harrigan, R.A., & Brady, W.J. (1999). ECG abnormalities in tricyclic antidepressant ingestion. *American Journal of Emergency Medicine, 17*, 387–393.

Hill, S.L., Evangelista, J.K., Pizzi, A.M., Mobassaleh, M., Fulton, D.R., & Berul, C.I. (1998). Proarrhythmia associated with Cisapride in children. *Pediatrics, 101*, 1053–1056.

Mishra, A., Friedman, H.S., & Sinha, A.K. (1999). The effects of erythromycin on the electrocardiogram. *Chest, 115*, 983–986.

Morganroth, J., & Goin, J.E. (1991). Quinidine-related mortality in the short-to-medium-term treatment of ventricular arrhythmias. A meta-analysis. *Circulation, 84*, 1977.

Morganroth, J., Talbot, G.H., Dorr, M.B., Johnson, R.D., Geary, W., and Magner, D. (1999). Effect of single ascending, supratherapeutic doses of sparfloxacin on cardiac repolarization (QTc interval). *Clinical Therapy, 21*, 818–828.

Warner, J.P., Barnes, T.R., & Henry, J.A. (1996). Electrocardiographic changes in patients receiving neuroleptic medications. *Acta Psychiactrica Scandinavica, 93*, 311–313.

# Chapter 5
# Sinus Rhythm and Sinus Arrhythmias
..................................................................

Normally, the heart will depolarize spontaneously and rhythmically. The rate will be controlled by the pacemaker that depolarizes at the fastest rate. The sinus node (SA node) normally has the highest frequency of discharge. Subsequent depolarization of atrial tissue will write a P wave on the ECG. If the impulse succeeds in traveling through the A-V junctions and activating the ventricles, a normal QRS complex (0.10 second) will follow. Variations in the sinus mechanisms have to do with rate and rhythm. As long as the sinus fires and atrial tissue responds, the process recurs normally at a given rate of speed. The clue is to look to the left of every QRS and find a single, positive P wave for each and every normal QRS—that is the sinus mechanism.

Consistent, step-by-step analysis is critical. Start by recognizing the normal wave forms and measurements and know what they reflect within the heart. Recognize any deviation, then correlate with physical findings, patient history, and medication or drug history.

Gathering information is the basis for a care plan, and each decision carries a grave responsibility. Choices of interventions are directed by a rapidly changing body of knowledge based on clinical research and governed by local and institutional protocols, and each intervention carries implications for risk versus relief.

## ARRHYTHMIAS ORIGINATING IN THE SA NODE

- Sinus bradycardia
- Sinus tachycardia
- Sinus arrhythmia
- Sinus arrest
- Sinus exit block

63

**Common Features of Sinus Mechanisms**

- Upright P waves in Leads I, II, III
- Similar appearance in all wave forms
- One (+) P for every QRS
- P-R interval 0.12 to 0.20 second
- QRS duration 0.10 second or less

## Approach to Interpretation

1. Plot P waves, calculating rate and rhythm.
2. Plot QRS complexes, calculating rate and rhythm.
3. Confirm the association between each P wave and the QRS complex.
4. Determine if the rhythm is appropriate to the patient.
5. Interpret the configuration and morphology using more than one ECG lead.
6. Select the appropriate intervention.

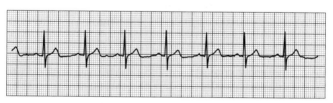

**Figure 5-1** Sinus rhythm.

**Characteristics of Sinus Rhythm**

- P waves are upright and normal and appear only before each QRS
- P-R interval is between 0.12 and 0.20 second and constant
- QRS complexes: 0.10 second

*continues*

*continued*
- Rate: between 60 and 100/minute
- Rhythm: essentially regular (see Figure 5-1)

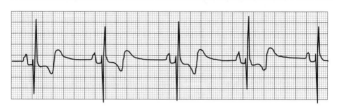

**Figure 5-2** Sinus bradycardia.

## Sinus Bradycardia

Sinus bradycardia (rate <60/minute) results from slowing of the SA node (see Figure 5-2).

### Possible Causes

- Increased parasympathetic tone
- Intrinsic SA node disease
- Right coronary artery disease
- Drug effects (digoxin, propranolol, quinidine)

### ECG Characteristics

- P waves: Upright, normal
- P-R interval: 0.12 to 0.20 second and constant
- QRS complex: 0.10 second or less
  - Rate: <60/minute
  - Rhythm: Regular

### Clinical Significance

Sinus bradycardia can result in decreased cardiac output, hypotension, angina, ventricular ectopics, lowering ventricular threshold, and ventricular arrhythmias.

### Proposed Interventions

1. Be supportive. If the patient is symptomatic, hypotensive and hyperperfusing, assess ABCs, oxygen ($O_2$), communicate with a physician (P), IV, history of present illness (HPI), chief complaint (CC), ?chest pain, ?meds, ?medical history (med Hx), ?vital signs, and ?allergies.
2. Detailed physical examination: Look for signs and symptoms (s/s) of congestive heart failure to include heart tones ($S_3$), peripheral edema, lung sounds (adventitious sounds), shortness of breath (SOB), and hypotension/hyperfusion (H/H).
3. Be alert for ectopy.
4. Consider medications to increase heart rate such as atropine 0.5 mg IV bolus, repeated every 3 to 5 minutes (3 mg or 0.04 mg/kg max).
5. Consider fluids.
6. Consider a vasopressor such as dopamine 2.5 to 10 µg/kg/minute for perfusion.
7. Consider a transcutaneous pacemaker.

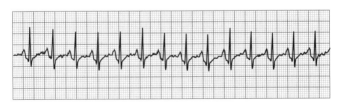

**Figure 5-3**  Sinus tachycardia.

### Sinus Tachycardia

Sinus tachycardia (rate >100/minute) results from increased sinus node discharge (see Figure 5-3).

### Possible Causes

- Cardiac failure
- Exercise

- Fever
- Hypovolemia, dehydration
- Increased sympathetic tone
- Pain, anxiety, anger

---

### ECG Characteristics
- P waves: Upright, normal
- P-R interval: 0.12 to 0.20 second and constant
- QRS complex: 0.10 second or less
  - Rate: >100/minute
  - Rhythm: Regular

---

### Clinical Significance
- Compensatory mechanism for decreased stroke volume as with CHF.
- As the rate increases, cardiac output may decrease and myocardial oxygen debt may increase.
- Can precipitate myocardial ischemia or infarct.
- Suggestive of cardiogenic shock if sustained with AMI.

### Proposed Interventions
1. Be supportive. If the patient is symptomatic, assess ABCs, $O_2$ , (P), IV, CC, ?chest pain, ?meds, ?medical history, ?vital signs, and ?allergies
2. Detailed physical examination: Look for s/s congestive heart failure to include heart tones ($S_3$), peripheral edema, lung sounds (adventitious sounds), SOB, and H/H.
3. Treat the underlying causes such as hypovolemia, pain, fever, anxiety, anger, CHF, and side effects to some medications. Administer prescribed antidote/interventions, for example, for illicit drugs.

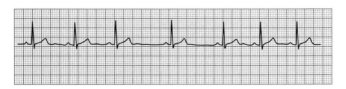

**Figure 5-4** Sinus arrhythmia.

### Sinus Arrhythmia

Sinus arrhythmia is characterized by a "regular irregularity," a gradual slowing then gradual increase in rate.

#### Possible Causes

- Related to respiratory cycle
- Can be caused by enhanced vagal tone

#### ECG Characteristics

- Pacemaker site: SA node
- P waves: Upright, normal
- P-R interval: 0.12 to 0.20 second
- QRS complex: ≤ 0.10 second
  - Rate: 60 to 100/minute
  - Rhythm: Irregular

#### Clinical Significance

Usually none.

#### Proposed Interventions

1. The patient is rarely symptomatic. If so, assess ABCs, s/s of H/H, $O_2$, (P), IV, HPI, CC, ?chest pain, ?meds, ?medical history, ?vital signs, and ?allergies
2. Detailed physical examination: as detailed as necessary based on CC and HP.
3. Be supportive.

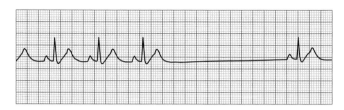

**Figure 5-5** Sinus rhythm > Sinus arrest 2.8 second.

### Sinus Arrest

Sinus arrest results from failure of the SA node to fire. There is no pattern of occurrence, and the arrest period is preceded and followed by sinus rhythm, bradycardia, or arrhythmia. The length of the arrest period may vary (see Figure 5-5).

#### Possible Causes

- SA node ischemia, right coronary artery disease
- Digitalis toxicity
- Excessive vagal tone
- Degenerative fibrotic disease

#### ECG Characteristics

- P waves: Upright, normal
- P-R interval: 0.12 to 0.20 second
- QRS complex: 0.10 second or less. There is a sudden drop of more than one PQRST complex.
  - Rate: Underlying rate 60 to 100/minute
  - Rhythm: Regular except for the arrest event *It is important to measure the duration of the arrest: the distance from the last QRS to the next QRS.* It is critical for the physician to know the precise length of the arrest period. Document the patient's signs and symptoms during this time.

### *Clinical Significance*

1. May decrease cardiac output, causing dizziness, sudden bouts of postural hypotension, and syncope.
2. May cause cardiac standstill.

### *Proposed Interventions*

Management when SA arrest persists and patient is symptomatic and H/H:

1. Assess ABCs, $O_2$, (P), IV, HPI, CC, ?chest pain, ?meds, ?medical history, ?vital signs, and ?allergies.
2. Detailed physical examination: s/s of H/H with the arrest periods. Question history (Hx) of near-syncopal episodes.
3. Consider medications to increase heart rate such as atropine 0.5 mg IV bolus, repeated every 3 to 5 minutes (up to 3.0 mg or 0.04 mg/kg max).
4. Consider IV fluids.
5. Consider a vasopressor such as dopamine 2.5 to 10 μg/kg/minute to increase perfusion.
6. Consider transcutaneous pacemaker.

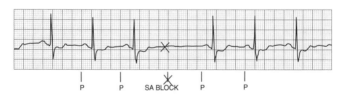

**Figure 5-6**   Sinus exit block.

### **Sinus Exit Block**

Sinus exit block is characterized by a sudden loss of one PQRST complex, usually resulting from atrial paralysis (see Figure 5-6).

### *Possible Causes*

• Drug induced, for example, quinidine.
• Normal variant (variation may occur without intrinsic pathology).

### ECG Characteristics

- P waves: Upright, normal
- P-R interval: 0.12 to 0.20 second
- QRS complex: 0.10 second or less—sudden drop of only one PQRST complex
  - Rate: underlying rate 60 to 100/minute
  - Rhythm: Regular except for the arrest event

### Clinical Significance

1. May decrease cardiac output, causing syncopal or near-syncopal episodes, dizziness, and postural hypotension.
2. May cause cardiac standstill.

### Proposed Interventions

Management of SA block is usually supportive. It is important to document medication history, because this is a probable cause. If the patient has an underlying bradycardia and is hypoperfusing, consider the following:

1. Assess ABCs, $O_2$, (P), IV, HPI, CC, ?chest pain, ?meds, ?medical history, ?vital signs, and ?allergies.
2. Detailed physical examination: assess for s/s congestive heart failure to include heart tones ($S_3$), peripheral edema, lung sounds (adventitious sounds), SOB, and H/H.
3. Consider medication to increase heart rate, such as atropine 0.5 mg IV bolus, repeated every 3 to 5 minutes (up to 3.0 mg or 0.04 mg/kg max).
4. Consider IV fluids.
5. Consider a vasopressor such as dopamine 2.5 to 10 µg/kg/minute for perfusion.
6. Consider a transcutaneous pacemaker.

## SUMMARY

Normally the sinus node dominates heart rhythm and does so for a lifetime. An arrhythmia is present when the heart rate is too slow, too fast, or irregular, or when depolarization does not propagate over atrial tissue and, finally, when the SA node fails to produce a stimulus at all.

Any change or deviation from normal should be assessed in terms of the situation in which it occurs. Consider whether the arrhythmia reflects an appropriate response or a sign of distinct pathology.

## REFERENCES

Glassman, A.H., et al. (1998). Cardiovascular effects of anti-depressant drugs. *Int Clin Psychopharmacol*, 13 Suppl 5, s25–30.

# Chapter 6
# Junctional Rhythm and
# Junctional Arrhythmias
...........................................................

Junctional beats originate from the AV junction, in the bundle of His, and can be escape (late), ectopic, or premature. The hallmark of the junctional mechanism is the negative P′ that occurs when there is retrograde conduction to the atria.

## ARRHYTHMIAS ORIGINATING IN THE AV JUNCTION

- Premature junctional complexes
- Junctional escape beats
- Idiojunctional rhythm
- Accelerated junctional rhythm
- Paroxysmal junctional tachycardia

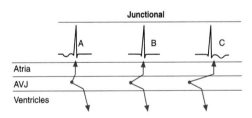

**Figure 6-1** Junctional induced complexes.

---

### Common Features of Junctional Mechanisms

- Inverted P′ waves
- (–)P′ waves may precede or follow QRS complex

*continues*

---

*continued*

- P′ waves may be absent
- P′-R interval less than 0.12 second
- QRS duration ≤ 0.10 second

## Approach to Interpretation

1. Plot out the sinus P waves if they are present, calculating rate and rhythm; if there are ectopics, determine if the sinus P plots through the ectopic event.
2. If no P waves occur before the QRS, plot out QRS rate and rhythm.
3. Determine if the junctional P′ is buried within the ST segment or T wave.

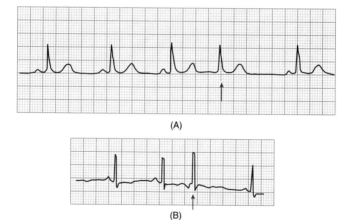

(A)

(B)

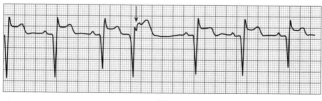

(C)

**Figure 6-2** Examples of junctional induced complexes.

## Premature Junctional Complexes (PJCs)

PJCs result from enhanced automaticity arising from the AV junction. When the PJC discharges a current, it may or may not conduct in a retrograde fashion to the atria. If it does, the resulting P′ will be negative and will occur before, during, or after the QRS complex (see Figure 6-2).

Successful retrograde conduction depends on the status and rate of speed of the anterograde and retrograde conduction pathways in the AV node.  The QRS is usually similar to the sinus-induced QRS since normal ventricular conduction is usually the case.

### Possible Causes

- Caffeine, tobacco, alcohol
- Digitalis
- Sympathomimetic drugs
- Ischemic heart disease, especially in acute inferior wall MI
- Hypoxia
- Rheumatic fever
- Normal variant

### ECG Characteristics

- P′ waves: May be present or not; negative wave form
- P′-R interval: About 0.12 second
- QRS complex: 0.10 second or less
  - Rate: Sinus rate calculated as the underlying rate
  - Rhythm: As is the underlying sinus rhythm

### Clinical Significance

Before deciding that isolated PJCs may be insignificant, consider the cause. If MI is suspected, the hemodynamic response to the underlying rhythm may be a critical issue. Treat the patient with a significant bradycardia or tachycardia as necessary.

If the patient is taking a digitalis preparation, assess for non-cardiac signs and symptoms of digitalis toxicity, such as anorexia, nausea, vomiting, blurred vision, arthralgia, color distortion and other vision disturbances, AV block, sinus bradycardia, PACs, PVCs, and ventricular bigeminy. Confirm with laboratory analysis as soon as possible.

### Proposed Interventions

1. Be supportive. If the patient is symptomatic, hypotensive, and hypoperfusing, assess ABCs, O$_2$, (P), and consider IV infusion.
2. Physical assessment and history: Assess HPI, CC, ?chest pain, ?med Hx, and ?meds (specifically digitalis).
3. If s/s of H/H with an underlying bradycardia, treat the bradycardia. PJCs are not treated.
4. If s/s of H/H with an underlying tachycardia, treat the tachycardia.
5. Serum electrolytes and digitalis levels should be assessed. However, therapeutic levels of digitalis do not rule out toxicity. PJCs are one of the first signs.

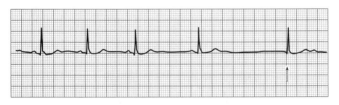

(A)

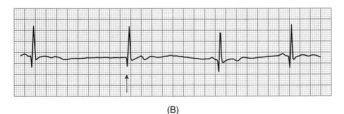

(B)

**Figure 6-3** Junctional escape beats.

## Junctional Escape Beats

Junctional escape beats result from long delays in the cardiac cycle. Where there is a bradycardia or a post-extra systolic pause (PAC, PVC), an impulse will discharge from the bundle of His within the AV junction. As with a PJC, the escape beat may or may not conduct in a retrograde fashion to the atria. If it does, the resulting P′ will be negative and will occur before, during, or after the QRS complex (see Figure 6-3).

The QRS is usually similar to the sinus-induced QRS since normal ventricular conduction is usually the case.

### Possible Causes

- Bradycardia
- Digitalis toxicity
- Hypoxia
- Ischemic heart disease; acute inferior wall MI
- Normal variant
- Post-extra systolic pause (common)
- Sympathomimetic drugs

### ECG Characteristics

- P′ waves: May be present or not; negative wave form
- P′-R interval: Usually 0.12 second
- QRS complex: 0.10 second or less
  - Rate: Sinus rate calculated as the underlying rate
  - Rhythm: As is the underlying sinus
- Occurs in sinus bradycardia or after a pause with SA block, SA arrest, PACs or PVCs

### Clinical Significance

Treat the patient who is symptomatic because of the bradycardia or, if known, the cause of the PAC or PVC.

### *Proposed Interventions*

1. If the patient is symptomatic, hypotensive, and hypoperfusing, be supportive: Assess ABCs, O$_2$, (P), and consider IV infusion.
2. Physical assessment and history: Assess HPI, CC, ?chest pain, ?med Hx, and ?meds (specifically digitalis).
3. If s/s of H/H with an underlying bradycardia, treat the bradycardia. Junctional escape beats are not treated.

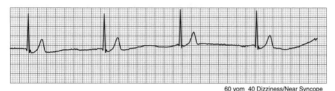

60 yom  40 Dizziness/Near Syncope

**Figure 6-4** Junctional rhythm.

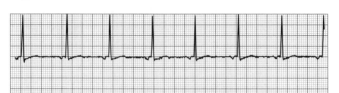

**Figure 6-5** Accelerated junctional rhythm.

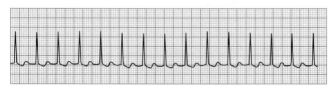

**Figure 6-6** Junctional tachycardia.

## Junctional and Idiojunctional Rhythm, Accelerated Junctional Rhythm, and Junctional Tachycardia

These variations of a junctional mechanism originate from the AV junction, in the bundle of His. Junctional tachycardia is an ectopic rhythm resulting from enhanced or triggered auto-maticity within the bundle of His. This ectopic controls ven-tricular rate.  The hallmark of the junctional mechanism is the negative P′ that occurs when there is retrograde conduction to the atria. If retrograde depolarization (negative P′) is intact, the prefix idio is not used. The difference between junctional rhythm, accelerated idiojunctional rhythm, and junctional tachycardia is rate (see Figures 6-4, 6-5, and 6-6).

### Possible Causes

- Abnormal automaticity with ischemia
- AV block
- Catecholamine surge
- Electrolyte imbalance
- Increased vagal tone
- Triggered automaticity with digitalis toxicity

### ECG Characteristics

- P′ waves: May be present or not; negative wave form
- P′-R interval: Usually 0.12 second
- QRS complex: 0.10 second or less
  - Rate: Junctional rhythm 40 to 60/minute
    Accelerated idiojunctional rhythm 60 to 100/minute
    Junctional tachycardia 100 to 140/minute
  - Rhythm: Regular

### Clinical Significance

Junctional rhythm and accelerated junctional rhythm may each occur as a protective mechanism with sinus arrest and profound sinus bradycardia.

### Proposed Interventions

1. Be supportive; Assess ABCs, O₂, (P), consider IV if s/s of H/H.
2. Physical assessment and history: Asses HPI, CC, ?chest pain, ?med Hx, and ?meds (specifically digitalis).

3. Serum electrolytes and digitalis levels should be assessed. However, therapeutic levels of digitalis do not rule out toxicity.

## SUMMARY

Junctional mechanisms occur primarily with ischemia and digitalis toxicity. The hallmark of this mechanism is the (−)P′ that may be seen before, during, or after the QRS complex. These rhythms as well as junctional escape complexes of themselves do not warrent intervention. The clinician should be alert to identifying the cause of junctional mechanisms.

# Chapter 7
# Atrial Ectopy and Atrial Arrhythmias

••••••••••••••••••••••••••••••••••••••••••••••••••••••••

The atrial mechanisms include PACs, tachycardias, atrial flutter, and atrial fibrillation and are often caused by physiological change, catecholamine surge, MI, and atrial stretch secondary to cardiac failure. In the setting of AMI, any sudden change in heart rate (i.e., atrial tachycardia, flutter, or fibrillation) can exacerbate the ischemia and injury and provoke ventricular ectopics, tachycardia, or fibrillation.

PACs (and PJCs) can initiate AV nodal reentry, resulting in paroxysmal supraventricular tachycardia. The clue to identification begins with plotting the sinus P waves.

## ARRHYTHMIAS ORIGINATING WITHIN THE ATRIA

- Premature atrial complexes and atrial bigeminy
- Paroxysmal atrial tachycardia (PAT) and paroxysmal supraventricular tachycardia (PSVT) with AV nodal reentry
- Atrial flutter
- Atrial fibrillation
- Atrial flutter with junctional escape rhythm
- Atrial fibrillation with junctional escape rhythm

### Common Features

- P′ waves often differ in size and amplitude from sinus P waves.
- P′-R interval may be shortened, prolonged, or normal.
- QRS duration is usually normal.
- PACs may or may not conduct to the ventricles.

## Approach to Interpretation

1. Plot the sinus P waves, calculating rate and rhythm. If there is an ectopic, determine if the sinus P wave plots through the ectopic event. If the sinus P wave cadence is disturbed, this may be caused by premature atrial depolarization.

2. If a normal QRS ectopic is followed by a pause, look to the left of the ectopic and determine if there is a premature (+) P wave just before or buried in the preceding T wave. This is the premature, ectopic atrial P wave.

3. If there is no ectopic yet a pause in the R-R interval, and the sinus cadence is disturbed, look to the left of the ectopic and determine if there is a premature (+) P wave just before or buried in the preceding T wave. This is the premature, ectopic atrial P wave that was unable to conduct into ventricular tissue, that is, a *nonconducted PAC*.

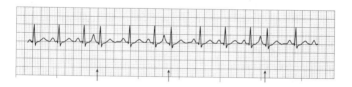

**Figure 7-1** Example of PACs.

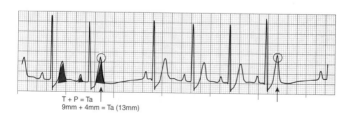

T + P = Ta
9mm + 4mm = Ta (13mm)

**Figure 7-2** Example of additive influence of P′ on T waves.

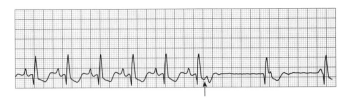

**Figure 7-3**   Example of nonconducted PAC.

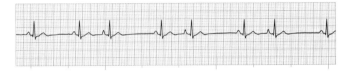

**Figure 7-4**   Atrial bigeminy.

## Premature Atrial Complex (PAC)

PACs result from single ectopic focus originating from within the atria. The P of the PAC is called a P prime (P′). The premature atrial depolarization often resets the sinus node so that the sinus P waves do not plot through the event (the PAC). After the PAC, the sinus cadence usually resumes. This is called *less than compensatory pause.* Occasionally the sinus node will be suppressed and the sinus cadence after the PAC will be slower. This is caused by *overdrive suppression* and usually does not persist (see Figures 7-1 through 7-4).

### Possible Causes

- Atrial stretch
- Caffeine, tobacco, alcohol
- CHF with MI
- Digitalis toxicity
- Electrolyte imbalance
- Emotional stress
- Hypertrophy
- Hypoxia

- No apparent cause (normal variant)
- Septal defects, valvular disease
- Sympathomimetic drugs

---

### ECG Characteristics

- P′ waves: Premature and different from sinus-induced P waves; (+) in leads I, II, aVF, $V_4$, and $V_6$. P′ waves may be easily identified as a nonconducted PAC and will often distort the T wave and cause an unexpected pause. Nonconducted PACs often add to the amplitude of the T wave on which they occur (additive influence). This is called the *Ta distortion*. Calculate the amplitude of a sinus P and add that to the amplitude of the normal T wave. That sum should equal the amplitude of the P′-on-T wave, the Ta (Figure 7-2).
- P′-R interval: The conducted PAC usually causes a P′-R that varies from sinus-induced P-R interval.
- QRS complex: 0.10 second or less or may be absent (nonconducted PAC). May be <0.10 second because of preexisting or rate-related bundle branch block or aberrant ventricular conduction.
  - Rate: As with the underlying rhythm.
  - Rhythm: Regular (as with sinus) except for the PAC. With atrial bigeminy, every other PQRST is premature.

---

### Clinical Significance

Isolated PACs must be assessed in the clinical situation where they appear. They may be of no consequence, but frequent PACs may indicate heart disease or CHF and may provoke an atrial tachycardia.

In the patient with chest pain, the catecholamine release with apprehension, anxiety, and fear can trigger a PAC. When this is the case, the PACs may relent with pain relief or sedation. However, if there is MI and the patient presents with sinus tachycardia and PACs or atrial bigeminy, the patient should be assessed for s/s of CHF. Bigeminal nonconducted PACs can cause a bradycardia that may cause hemodynamic compromise.

### Proposed Interventions

1. If the patient is asymptomatic, be supportive.
2. If symptomatic, hypotensive, and hypoperfusing, assess ABCs, $O_2$, (P), and consider IV infusion.
3. Physical assessment and history: Assess HPI, CC, ?chest pain, ?med Hx, and ?meds (specifically digitalis). Assess for s/s of CHF including peripheral edema and heart sounds for $S_3$.
4. If s/s of H/H with an underlying bradycardia, treat the bradycardia. PACs are not treated.
5. If s/s of H/H with an underlying tachycardia, treat the tachycardia and assess for s/s of CHF as in item 3.
6. Serum electrolytes and digitalis levels should be assessed. However, therapeutic levels of digitalis may not rule out toxicity.

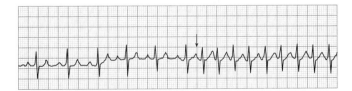

**Figure 7-5**   Sinus → PAC → atrial tachycardia.

## Supraventricular Tachycardias (PAT and PSVT)

PAT results from sudden onset of rapid atrial depolarization overriding the SA node at a rate range of 130 to 250/minute. The natural tendency of the AV node is to deter conduction; the faster the rate of discharge from the atrial ectopic, the greater the AV delay. However, the AV node can sustain the

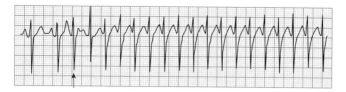

**Figure 7-6**   Sinus → PAC and resulting tachycardia.

tachycardia by an AV nodal reentry mechanism (see Figures 7-5 and 7-6).

*Reentry* is defined as the ability of an impulse to reexcite some region of the atria through which it has already passed. Reentry usually occurs when an impulse deviates into a circular conduction pathway, forming a loop. There are dual pathways in the AV node of differing conduction rates and refractory levels, which, when activated separately, support a reentrant tachycardia.

### Possible Causes

- Digitalis toxicity
- Heart disease
- Sometimes accompanied by Wolff Parkinson White (WPW) syndrome
- Stress, smoking, overexertion, caffeine

### ECG Characteristics

- Pacemaker site: Atrial ectopic focus.
- P′ waves: Cannot be clearly delineated because of the rapid rate. P′ wave forms may be seen with the QRS complex or may be seen distorting the end of the QRS that may look like broad, terminal S waves as seen in RBBB.
- P′-R interval: May not be possible to differentiate P′ from the T wave in most instances. Look for prolonged P′-R interval just before the tachycardia.

*continues*

*continued*

- QRS complex: 0.10 second or less; >0.10 second when there is preexisting or rate-related bundle branch block. Aberrant ventricular conduction is rare with PSVT with AV nodal reentry. Observe for QRS alternans (alternating QRS heights or depths). Once the PSVT with AV nodal reentry is established, there is usually no alternans. If QRS alternans is present, circus movement tachycardia must be suspected.
  - Rate: 150 to 180+/minute; with PSVT the rate can reach 250+.
  - Rhythm: Regular.
  **The hallmarks of a PAT and PSVT are the sudden onset and rapid, regular rhythm.**

## Clinical Significance of Atrial Tachycardia

Atrial tachycardia may deteriorate into atrial flutter or fibrillation. The rapid rate diminishes cardiac output and decreases coronary artery perfusion, which, in turn, may precipitate angina, hypotension, CHF, ventricular tachycardia, or fibrillation.

## Proposed Interventions

1. If the patient is asymptomatic, be supportive. If hypotensive and hypoperfusing, assess ABCs, $O_2$, (P), and consider IV infusion.
2. Physical assessment and history: Assess HPI, CC, ?chest pain, ?med Hx, and ?meds (specifically digitalis). Assess for s/s of CHF including peripheral edema and heart sounds for $S_3$. The patient may report feeling palpitations, dizziness, lightheadedness, full sensation in the neck, ringing in the ears, and unexplained anxiety.
3. Assess serum electrolytes and digitalis levels.
4. Consider vagal maneuvers (Valsalva, carotid sinus massage). However, this may not interrupt the tachy-

cardia. In the case of a PAT, if such a maneuver does interrupt the tachycardia, the PAT may recur. Vagal maneuvers may help differentiate sinus tachycardia from atrial tachycardias, because with a sinus mechanism there would be a gradual slowing during the maneuver.

5. Consider medications to delay conduction in the AV node such as adenosine 6 mg IV bolus, which may be repeated.
6. If adenosine fails to convert, consider verapamil 5 mg IV bolus, which may be repeated.
7. If the patient is unstable, prepare for synchronized cardioversion.
8. Consider sedation before cardioversion.

### *Clinical Significance of PAT/PSVT*

The patient may sense palpitations, dizziness, lightheadedness, or anxiety, or PAT/PSVT may cause serious deterioration in perfusion so the patient has altered level of consciousness. In a patient who is of advanced age or who has cardiac disease, the rapid ventricular rate may further compromise cardiac output, which may precipitate angina, hypotension, CHF, ventricular tachycardia, and fibrillation.

### *Proposed Interventions*

1. If there is H/H, assess ABCs, $O_2$, (P), and consider IV infusion; if there is altered level of consciousness (ALOC), prepare for immediate synchronized cardioversion.
2. Physical assessment and history: Assess HPI and CC, ?chest pain, ?med Hx, and ?meds (specifically digitalis). Assess for s/s of CHF including peripheral edema and heart sounds for $S_3$. The patient may report feeling palpitations, dizziness, lightheadedness, full sensation in the neck, ringing in the ears, and unexplained anxiety.
3. Serum electrolytes and digitalis levels should be assessed. However, therapeutic levels of digitalis do not rule out toxicity.

4. Consider vagal maneuvers (Valsalva, carotid sinus massage). However, this may not interrupt the tachycardia, or if it does, the PSVT may recur.
5. Consider adenosine 6 mg IV bolus, which may be repeated.
6. If adenosine fails to convert, consider verapamil 2.5 to 5 mg IV bolus, which may be repeated.
7. If unstable, prepare for synchronized cardioversion.
8. Consider sedation before cardioversion.

## Atrial Flutter

Atrial flutter is a macroreentrant trachyarrhythmia most often contained within the right atrium. Atrial flutter is thought to result from an atrial ectopic often contained in the right atrium and sustained with a rapid atrial reentry circuit. Therapeutic delay at the AV node will prevent many of the atrial impulses from conducting through to the ventricles. The ventricular response can be regular or irregular.

Atrial flutter is not considered a normal variant and is seen in patients with myocardial ischemia and may cause reentrant tachycardias. New electrocardiographic criteria are being developed for the differentiation between counterclockwise and clockwise atrial flutter through correlation with electrophysiological study and radiofrequency catheter ablation. Its clinical significance remains to be defined.

### Possible Causes
- Atrial stretch from acute illness
- Heart disease

### ECG Characteristics
- Atrial = flutter waves at 250 to 300/minute.
- Rhythm: Regular or irregular.
- Pacemaker site: Atrial ectopic focus.

*continues*

*continued*

- P waves: Flutter waves sometimes referred to as "saw-tooth" or "picket fence." They can be plotted out more easily on the negative component.
- P′-R interval: Constant but will vary with irregular ventricular response. The flutter wave (P′) immediately preceding the QRS is not necessarily the wave front directly responsible for the QRS. It is impossible to determine specificity of conduction without His-bundle ECG analysis.
  - Rate: Varies.
  - Complex: 0.10 second or less (may be distortion from atrial flutter waves).
- T wave may be distorted at the baseline because of the flutter waves (referred to as Ta distortion).

### Clinical Significance

The presence of atrial flutter may be the first indication of cardiac disease. In the setting of rapid ventricular rates, cardiac output may be decreased.

### Proposed Interventions

1. If there is H/H, assess ABCs, $O_2$, (P), and consider IV infusion. If there is ALOC, prepare for immediate synchronized cardioversion.
2. Physical assessment and history: Assess HPI, CC, ?chest pain, ?med Hx, and ?meds. Assess for evidence of heart disease including those associated with CHF. The patient may report sudden rapid heart rate, dizziness, a thumping in the chest, and lightheadedness.
3. Consider current pharmacological interventions. Consider calcium-channel blockers such as verapamil 2.5 to 5 mg IV bolus, which may be repeated.
4. Consider rate-controlling medications such as digitalis and diltiazem.

5. Consider beta-blockers.
6. Consider antiarrhythmics such as procainamide.
7. If the patient is unstable, synchronized cardioversion may be necessary.
8. Consider sedation before synchronized cardioversion

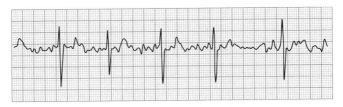

**Figure 7-7**   Atrial fibrillation.

## Atrial Fibrillation

The true origin of atrial fibrillation is unknown, but it is thought to result from multiple reentry areas within atria. Characteristically, there is a random, irregular ventricular response. There is no organized atrial contraction, and atrial kick is lost. The onset of atrial fibrillation is accompanied by a rapid irregular rate, which may cause deterioration from myocardial ischemia (see Figure 7-7).

### Possible Causes

- Atherosclerotic heart disease
- Atrial dilation
- Caffeine
- Cocaine
- Congestive heart failure
- Digitalis toxicity
- ETOH
- Hyperthyroidism, Age, Hypertension
- Long-term chronic lung disease, chronic renal and hepatic disease
- Rheumatic heart disease
- Thyrotoxicosis

*ECG Characteristics*
- Atrial rate 350 to 750 (usually unable to verify)
- Pacemaker site: Atrial tissue
- P′ waves: None, chaotic baseline
- P′-R interval: Not applicable
    - QRS complex: 0.10 second or less unless there is rate-related or preexisting bundle branch block
    - Rate: Irregular

## Clinical Significance

As with atrial flutter, atrial fibrillation can compromise cardiac output as much as 20 to 25%, resulting in H/H, CHF, and cardiogenic shock. Pulse deficits are noted on examination of all extremities. The major morbidity from atrial fibrillation is arterial emboli from thrombus formation in the atrial chamber resulting in pulmonary or cerebral emboli.

The sudden onset of atrial fibrillation may decrease cardiac output, possibly acutely. The rhythm may convert spontaneously within a few hours without intervention.

If the patient shows signs of hemodynamic compromise, assess the ECG for signs of myocardial ischemia: ST elevation or depression, inverted T waves, and the appearance of Q waves.

## Proposed Interventions

1. If there is H/H, assess ABCs, $O_2$, (P), and consider IV infusion. If there is ALOC, prepare for immediate synchronized cardioversion.
2. Physical assessment and history: Assess HPI and CC, ?chest pain, ?med Hx, and ?meds. Assess for evidence of heart disease including those associated with CHF. The patient may report sudden rapid heart rate, dizziness, a thumping in the chest, lightheadedness, and dyspnea.
3. Consider current pharmacological medications for conversion. Consider calcium-channel blockers such as verapamil 2.5 to 5 mg IV bolus, which may be repeated.

4. Consider beta-blockers, diltiazem or digitalis, procainamide, quinidine.
5. If the patient is unstable, prepare for synchronized cardioversion.
6. Consider sedation before cardioversion.

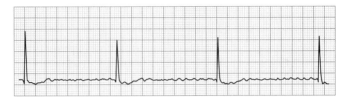

**Figure 7-8**   Atrial fibrillation, junctional escape rhythm.

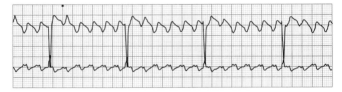

**Figure 7-9**   Atrial flutter, junctional escape rhythm.

### Atrial Flutter and Fibrillation with Junctional Escape Rhythm

Atrial flutter can have regular or irregular ventricular rhythm; atrial fibrillation should only have irregular ventricular response. If the rhythm is regular and slow, AV block due to digitalis is almost always the cause, and the use of a vagolytic medication such as atropine may not be used and electronic pacing is preferred (see Figures 7-8 and 7-9).

### *Possible Causes*

Atrial flutter and fibrillation with junctional rhythm associated with AV block is usually induced by digitalis. There may be group beating, PVCs, and ventricular bigeminy.

*ECG Characteristics*

- P waves: None.
  Atrial flutter sawtooth waves at 250 to 300/minute.
  Atrial fibrillation at rates unable to be determined.
- Pacemaker site: Atrial focus, but the focus for the ventricular rate is from the AV junction.
- P'-R interval: Constant but will vary with irregular ventricular response.
- QRS complex: 0.10 second or less (may not appear consistent in duration and amplitude due to distortion from atrial fibrillation and flutter waves).
  - Rate: >70/minute.
  - Rhythm: Very regular.

*Clinical Significance*

The patient is usually symptomatic with the digitalis toxicity and resulting bradycardia. Furthermore, the atria do not contribute to cardiac output, and risk of mural emboli is great.

*Proposed Interventions*

1. If there are H/H and ALOC, assess ABCs, $O_2$, (P), and consider IV infusion. Prepare for transcutaneous or transvenous pacing as soon as possible.
2. Physical assessment and history: Assess HPI, CC, ?chest pain, ?med Hx, and ?meds, especially for digitalis preparations. Assess for s/s digitalis toxicity, and confirm with laboratory analysis as soon as possible.
3. Consider digoxin immune fab (Digibind®), an antibody to digitalis via bolus, or IV infusion dependent on patient condition.
4. May sedate during transcutaneous pacing.

## SUMMARY

The atrial mechanisms consist of ectopic complexes and arrhythmias that primarily occur with cardiac disease. They range from single ectopics, to reentry mechanisms within the atria or the AV node. There is a wide variety of patient presentation, from new-onset to chronic or repetitive atrial arrhythmias. Each occurrence must be assessed within the patient's clinical presentation. Assessment and history are critical in formulating an effective care plan.

## REFERENCES

Daoud, E.G., & Morady, F. (1998). Pathophysiology of atrial flutter. *Annual Revue of Medicine, 49*, 77–83.

Lai, L.P., Lin, J.L., Lin, L.J., Chen, W.J., Ho, Y.L., Tseng, Y.Z., Chen, C.H., Lee, Y.T., Lien, W.P., and Huang, S.K. (1998). New electrocardiographic criteria for the differentiation between counterclockwise and clockwise atrial flutter: correlation with electrophysiological study and radiofrequency catheter ablation. *Heart, 80*, 80–85.

Roithinger, F.X., & Lesh, M.D. (1999). What is the relationship of atrial flutter and fibrillation? *Pacing Clinical Electrophysiology, 22*, 643–654.

# Chapter 8
# Ventricular Ectopy, Ventricular Arrhythmias, Asystole, and Pulseless Electrical Activity

Ventricular ectopy is the result of altered automaticity, after-depolarization, or reentry. Ventricular mechanisms include idioventricular rhythm and accelerated ventricular rhythm, ventricular tachycardia, and fibrillation. Ventricular ectopics are named for where they occur within the cardiac cycle.

Asystole and pulseless electrical activity are conditions that must be confirmed by patient assessment and, in the case of asystole, by visualization and comparison of various ECG leads.

## ARRHYTHMIAS ORIGINATING IN THE VENTRICLES

- Idioventricular rhythm, accelerated idioventricular rhythm
- Premature ventricular complex (PVC)
  a. Uniform
  b. Multiform
  c. Paired (couplet)
  d. End-diastolic
  e. Interpolated
  f. R-on-T phenomenon
- *Runs* or *episodes* of ventricular tachycardia (three or more PVCs in succession)
- Sustained ventricular tachycardia
- Torsade de pointes
- Ventricular fibrillation
- Aberrant ventricular conduction

### Common Features

- QRS of the ventricular complex is different from the underlying QRS.
- QRS complex is usually greater than 0.10 second. The impulse arises within ventricular tissue and does not use the bundle branch system.
- QRS is opposite in polarity to its T wave.
  a.  QRS (+) – T (–)
  b.  QRS (–) – T (+)

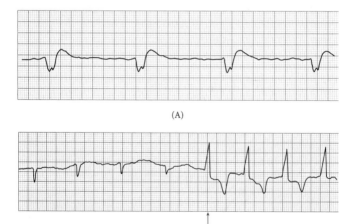

(A)

(B)

**Figure 8-1**  (A) Idioventricular rhythm. (B) Accelerated ventricular rhythm.

### Approach to Interpretation

Plot the sinus P waves, calculating rate and rhythm. If there is an ectopic, determine if the sinus P wave plots through the ectopic event. If the sinus P wave cadence is not disturbed, the ectopic is probably ventricular in origin.

## Ventricular Escape Complexes and Idioventricular Rhythm (IVR)

IVR appears in the presence of depressed or absent supraventricular pacing sites. The IVR focus in the ventricle begins pacing the heart as the last safety mechanism (see Figure 8-1).

### Possible Causes

- AV block
- Failed junctional escape mechanism
- Accelerated IVR may be seen in patient undergoing thrombolytic therapy as a reperfusion arrhythmia.

### ECG Characteristics

- P waves: Does not apply.
- P-R interval: Does not apply.
- QRS complex: Usually >0.10 with QRS/T wave opposite in polarity.

### Clinical Significance

The escape mechanism is not treated as an arrhythmia unless it is thought to be a competitive mechanism, as with AV dissociation. Diminished cardiac output is expected because of the slow rate.

### Proposed Interventions

Note: IVR should not be suppressed.

1. If the patient is symptomatic, hypotensive, or hypoperfusing, assess ABCs, O$_2$, (P), and IV infusion.
2. Physical assessment and history: Assess HPI, CC, ?chest pain, ?med Hx, ?meds, vital signs, and allergies.
3. If s/s of H/H with an underlying bradycardia, treat the bradycardia.

4. Consider medication currently accepted for increasing the rate, such as atropine 0.5 mg IV bolus, repeated in 3 to 5 minutes (up to 3.0 mg max or 0.04 mg/kg max) in an effort to reestablish a higher order of rhythm.
5. Consider fluids and vasopressor therapy such as dopamine for perfusion.
6. Consider transcutaneous pacing (may be the first intervention).

If patient is pulseless:

1. Begin CPR, assessing pulses with CPR. Ventilate 12 to 20/minute with 100% oxygen; intubate. Initiate current advanced cardiac life support protocols including epinephrine 1 mg IV bolus every 3 to 5 minutes.
2. Administer fluid challenge.
3. Initiate transcutaneous or transvenous pacing as soon as possible.
4. Consider cessation of efforts if no response and according to current clinical standards.

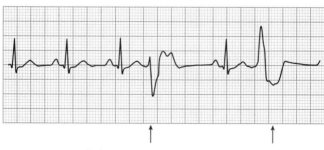

**Figure 8-2**  Multiform PVCs.

## Premature Ventricular Complex (PVC)

PVCs usually result from an ectopic focus arising from irritable ventricular focus, usually hypoxia-induced, and replace a normally expected QRS. PVCs may be unifocal or multifocal in origin. Shape and polarity alone do not guarantee that differentiation. More correct terms are *uniform* and *multiform* in appearance (see Figure 8-2).

PVCs may be coupled or may occur in various patterns (see Figure 8-3):

1. Bigeminy (every other beat) (see Figure 8-4).
2. Trigeminy (every third beat) (see Figure 8-5).
3. Quadrigeminy (every fourth beat).
4. R-on-T PVC may cause ventricular tachycardia or fibrillation if it falls on the vulnerable portion of the T wave (see Figure 8-6).

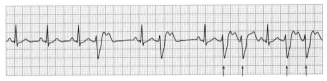

**Figure 8-3**   Paired PVCs or couplets.

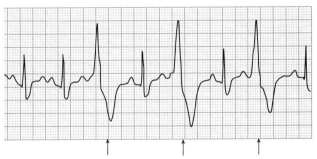

**Figure 8-4**   Ventricular bigeminy.

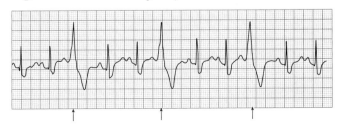

**Figure 8-5**   Ventricular trigeminy.

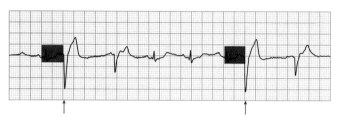

**Figure 8-6** R-on-T PVC.

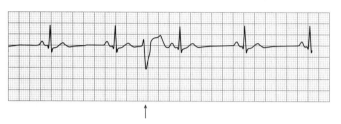

**Figure 8-7** Interpolated PVC.

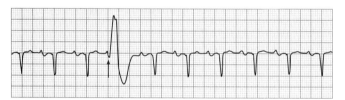

**Figure 8-8** End-diastolic PVC.

5. Interpolated: sandwiched between two normally occurring QRS complexes. As such, the interpolated PVC does not take the place of a normally occurring QRS (see Figure 8-7).
6. Frequent, multiformed.
7. Couplets or runs of VT (three or more in succession).

### Possible Causes

- Acid-base abnormalities
- Digitalis
- Electrolyte abnormalities

- Hypertension
- Hypovolemia
- Hypoxia
- Idiopathic
- Increased sympathetic tone
- Myocardial ischemia
- Rapid rates, insufficient to maintain adequate perfusion
- Slow rates, insufficient to maintain adequate perfusion
- Stress

### ECG Characteristics

- Pacemaker site: As with underlying rhythm.
- P waves: As with the underlying rhythm.
- P-R interval: As with the underlying rhythm.
- QRS Rate: As with the underlying rhythm.
- QRS complex: As with the underlying rhythm.
  a. QRS of the PVC is different.
  b. QRS/T wave polarity is opposite.
  c. Sinus P wave usually plots through.
  d. QRS duration is usually greater than 0.10 second.

### Clinical Significance

PVCs often indicate ventricular irritability in the patient with ischemia. Patients often sense "skipped beats."

### Proposed Interventions

1. If the patient is symptomatic, hypotensive, and hypo-perfusing, assess ABCs, $O_2$, (P), and IV infusion.
2. Physical assessment and history: Assess HPI and CC, ?chest pain, ?med Hx, ?meds (digitalis), vital signs, and allergies.
3. If s/s of H/H with an underlying bradycardia, treat the bradycardia.
4. Treat possible cardiac pain if present; administer nitroglycerin and morphine according to current protocol; reassess pain, blood pressure, and effect on the ectopy.

5. If PVCs persist or increase in frequency:
   a. Consider the appropriate antiarrhythmic therapy such as lidocaine 1 to 1.5 mg/kg IV bolus; repeat at 0.5 to 0.75 mg/kg IV bolus every 5 minutes until PVCs abate or 3 mg/kg has been given.
   b. Consider lidocaine drip at 3 to 4 mg/minute; 1 mg > total bolus dose.
   c. If patient is allergic or refractory to lidocaine, consider procainamide, bretylium, or amiodarone.

## Ventricular Tachycardia (VT)

VT is defined as three or more ventricular complexes in succession, with ventricular ectopic focus overriding the underlying rhythm. VT can occur in episodes or runs or can be the dominant rhythm, called *sustained VT.*

### Possible Causes

The possible causes of VT are the same as with PVCs, and its persistence is thought to be the result of a reentry circuit within ventricular tissue. Altered automaticity after depolarization is another probable cause (see Figure 8-9).

---

*ECG Characteristics of VT*

- Pacemaker: As with the underlying rhythm.
- P waves: As with the underlying rhythm.
- P-R interval: As with the underlying rhythm.
- QRS rate: As with underlying rhythm. The episodes of ventricular tachycardia are usually >100 per minute.
- QRS complex: As with the underlying rhythm.
  a. The QRS of the PVC is different.
  b. QRS/T wave polarity is opposite.
  c. Sinus P wave usually plots through.
  - Rate: sustained VT = 100 to 250/minute.
  - Rhythm: Regular.

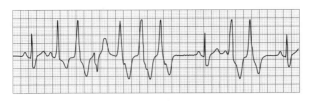

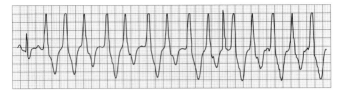

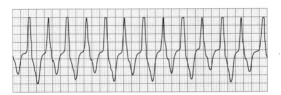

**Figure 8-9** Episodes of ventricular tachycardia progressing to sustained ventricular tachycardia.

### ECG Characteristics of Sustained VT

- Pacemaker site: Ventricular focus.
- P waves: Not always visible; depends on the rate of the VT.
- PR interval: Not applicable.
- QRS complex: >0.10 with QRS/T opposite polarity.
  a. $V_1$ shows a monophasic R wave, QR, qR, or RS, or twin peaks to the R wave, the first being taller (rabbit ear).
  b. Concordant negativity in precordial leads supports ventricular tachycardia.
  - Rate: >100 beats/minute.
  - Rhythm: Regular.
- Left axis deviation.

## *Clinical significance*

Sustained VT usually results in low cardiac output. The faster the rhythm, the less perfusion. It is critical to confirm the presence or absence of pulses, as the patient may be perfusing, poorly perfusing, or dead. Sustained VT may deteriorate to ventricular fibrillation or asystole.

## *Proposed Interventions*

If the patient with sustained VT is stable and perfusing:

1. H/H; assess ABCs, $O_2$, (P), and IV infusion.
2. Physical assessment and history: Assess HPI, CC, ?chest pain, ?med Hx, ?meds (digitalis), vital signs, and allergies.
3. Administer appropriate antiarrhythmic therapy such as lidocaine 1 to 1.5 mg/kg IV bolus; repeat at 0.5 to 0.75 mg/kg IV bolus every 5 minutes until conversion or until 3 mg/kg has been given.
4. If allergic or refractory to lidocaine, consider alternative medications such as procainamide, bretylium, or amiodrarone.

If patient is unstable (e.g., decreased LOC, hypotension), perform immediate synchronized cardioversion at 100 joules. If patient is pulseless, treat as ventricular fibrillation and defibrillate beginning at 200 joules.

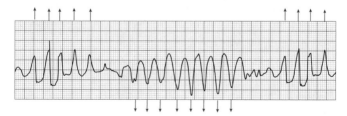

**Figure 8-10**   Torsade de pointes.

## Torsade de Pointes (TdP)

TdP is a term to describe the polymorphic nature of this form of ventricular tachycardia. TdP is usually associated with a prolonged QT interval and is thought to be caused by triggered automaticity. The QRS polarity reverses polarity, which is called by a French term meaning "twisting of the points" (see Figure 8-10).

### Possible Causes

- Antiarrhythmic medications such as quinidine, procainamide, disopyramide, or amiodarone
- Congenital heart disease
- Electrolyte imbalance, such as hypokalemia, hypocalcemia, and hypomagnesemia
- Profound bradycardia often with AV block
- Intracranial pathology such as subarachnoid hemorrhage or trauma
- Psychotropic drugs such as phenothiazine and tricylic antidepressants
- Organophosphate poisoning
- Prolonged QT interval (idiopathic)

### ECG Characteristics

TdP almost always begins with a prolonged QT interval and a long–short cardiac cycle. The phasic variations of the QRS complexes have no set length of time between twists.

- Pacemaker site: Ventricular focus.
- P waves: May be visible before or after the TdP. In sustained TdP, P waves are not visible.
- PR interval: Not applicable.
- QRS complex: >0.10 with QRS/T opposite polarity. Phasic variation in the polarity of the QRS complexes is sometimes described as a "spindle effect."
- Rate: 150 to 250, often unable to count.
- QT interval: Greater than one half the preceding R-R interval.
- Long–short R-R cycle prior to the tachycardia.

### Clinical Significance

TdP usually results in low cardiac output. The faster the rhythm, the less perfusion. It is critical to confirm pulses, to determine if the patient is perfusing adequately, poorly perfusing, or dead. TdP may deteriorate to ventricular fibrillation or asystole.

### Proposed Interventions

1. If the patient is stable and perfusing, assess ABCs, $O_2$, (P), and IV infusion.
2. Physical assessment, detailed physical exam, and focused history: Assess LOC, HPI, CC, ?chest pain, ?med Hx, ?meds (e.g., antiarrhythmic, recreational, psychotropic; see Possible Causes), vital signs, and allergies.
3. Magnesium Sulfate IV: push 2 g over 1 to 2 minutes; IV infusion 1 to 2 g/hour for 4 to 6 hours.
4. Perform temporary overdrive transcutaneous or transvenous pacing with sedation whenever possible.
5. If the patient is unstable (e.g., decreased LOC, hypotension), perform immediate defibrillation at 200 joules.
6. If the patient is pulseless, treat as ventricular fibrillation and defibrillate beginning at 200 joules.

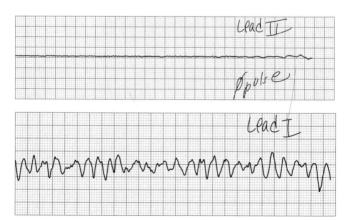

**Figure 8-11** Apparent asystole in lead II but confirmed as ventricular fibrillation in lead I.

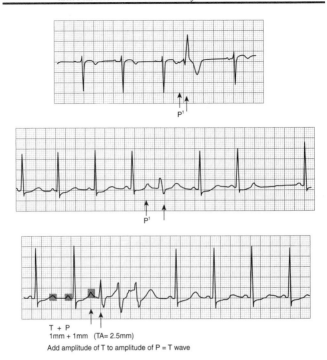

T + P
1mm + 1mm   (TA= 2.5mm)
Add amplitude of T to amplitude of P = T wave

**Figure 8-14**   Examples of PACs with aberrant ventricular conduction.

## Aberrant Ventricular Conduction

Aberrant ventricular conduction is really transient conduction problems within one or more of the bundle branches (see Figure 8-14).

### Possible Causes

- Preexisting bundle branch block
- Rate-dependent bundle branch block

### ECG Characteristics

- Pacemaker site: As with underlying rhythm
- P waves: As with underlying rhythm

*continues*

*continued*

- PR interval: As with underlying rhythm
- QRS complex: As with underlying rhythm except for the ectopic
  a. In a sinus rhythm, plot sinus P waves. If the cadence changes suddenly, look for P′ in the ST-T preceding the ectopic.
  b. Aberrant beats may show a triphasic rsR′ in $V_1$ and a triphasic qRs in $V_6$.
  c. No concordant negativity in precordial leads for the aberrant beats (be sure leads are simultaneous).
  - Rate: As with underlying rhythm except for sudden change in polarity of QRS
  - Rhythm: As with underlying rhythm except for sudden change

### Clinical Significance

A rule of thumb is that any QRS different from the normally occurring QRS is considered ventricular until proven otherwise. Whenever there is a sudden change in rate and the patient's presentation has not changed, the clinician should suspect aberration. Carefully compare previous tracings and any previous occurrence of ectopics, if available.

If supraventricular tachycardia (SVT) with aberrant conduction is suspected, whenever possible confirm with 12-lead ECG.

### Proposed Interventions

1. If the patient is symptomatic, hypotensive, and hypoperfusing, assess ABCs, $O_2$, (P), and IV infusion.
2. Physical assessment and history: Assess HPI, CC, ?chest pain, ?med Hx, ?meds, vital signs, and allergies.
3. If s/s of H/H with an underlying bradycardia, treat the bradycardia.
4. With sustained tachycardia, if the QRS morphology changes with sudden increase in heart rate, assess the patient and attempt to confirm the source with 12-lead ECG.

## Ventricular Fibrillation (VF)

VF is a chaotic ventricular discharge resulting from many reentry circuits but with no ventricular depolarization or contraction. The patient may display agonal breathing or jerking movements of the extremities, but there is no pulse and no cardiac output (see Figure 8-11).

### Possible Causes

- Advanced coronary artery disease
- R-on-T, frequent, paired, or multiformed PVCs in the setting of acute myocardial infarction
- Drug abuse
- Traumatic event
- Electrical injuries

### ECG Characteristics

- Rate: Not discernible
- Rhythm: Not discernible
- Pacemaker site: Numerous ectopic foci in ventricle
- P waves: None
- P-R interval: None
- QRS complex: None

### Clinical Significance

Rapid identification and defibrillation are critical in treating the patient with VF. The longer the delay in intervention, the less success in conversion to a higher order of rhythm.

### Proposed Interventions

1. Initiate CPR and manage the airway until a defibrillator is available.
2. Initiate advanced cardiac life support protocols including defibrillation as soon as possible.
3. Establish airway control, intubation, and IV access.

4.  Initiate advanced cardiac life support protocols such as epinephrine 1 mg IV bolus every 3 to 5 minutes.
5.  Defibrillate between medications according to protocol.
6.  Consider lidocaine, bretylium and amiodarone.

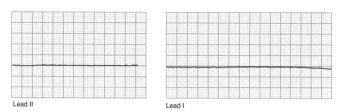

Lead II

Lead I

**Figure 8-12**  Asystole confirmed in a second lead.

## Asystole

Asystole implies absence of all cardiac activity (see Figure 8-12). In some instances, the atria continue to beat in their own time.

### Asystole vs. Fine Ventricular Fibrillation

Ventricular fibrillation is the result of chaotic activity within the ventricular system. Many fibers are depolarizing, and there is no effective perfusion. When the flow of current is largely parallel to the monitoring lead, the fibrillation is easily recognized. However, when the flow of current is at a right angle to the monitoring lead, the ECG may look like asystole. It is critical to switch from lead II to leads I and III to differentiate asystole from ventricular fibrillation.

### Possible Causes

*   Myocardial infarction
*   Traumatic event

- Hypoxia
- Electrolyte imbalance: hyperkalemia or hypokalemia
- Hypothermia
- Acid-base imbalance
- Drug overdose

*ECG Characteristics*

Note: Always confirm in at least one other lead!

- Rate: None
- Rhythm: None
- Pacemaker site: None
- P waves: None
- P-R interval: None
- QRS complex: None

*Clinical Significance*

In asystole, there is no cardiac output, and the prognosis for resuscitation is poor.

*Proposed Interventions*

1. Initiate CPR.
2. Establish airway control and IV access.
3. Initiate current advanced cardiac life support therapy including epinephrine 1 mg every 3 to 5 minutes during arrest.
4. Consider immediate transcutaneous pacing.
5. Consider atropine 1 mg IV bolus; may repeat every 3 to 5 minutes for a total of 3 mg.
6. Consider sodium bicarbonate depending on the patient's clinical situation.
7. Carefully evaluate the clinical situation before considering cessation of efforts.

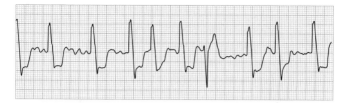

**Figure 8-13**   ECG tracing with pulseless electrical activity.

## Pulseless Electrical Activity (PEA)

PEA occurs when there is an identifiable rhythm but the patient is unresponsive and does not have a palpable pulse. The ECG rhythm may be sinus, atrial, or junctional in origin, or one of the AV conduction defects may be present (see Figure 8-13).

Despite the presence of electrical function (the ECG rhythm), there is no mechanical response, no cardiac output, no pulse, and no blood pressure.

### Possible Causes

- Acid-base imbalance
- Drug overdose
- Electrolyte imbalance: hyperkalemia
- Hypothermia
- Hypovolemia
- Hypoxia
- Myocardial infarction
- Pulmonary embolus
- Tension pneumothorax

### ECG Characteristics

- Rate: As with underlying rhythm
- Rhythm: As with underlying rhythm
- Pacemaker site: As with underlying rhythm
- P waves: As with underlying rhythm

*continues*

*continued*

- P-R interval: As with underlying rhythm
- QRS complex: As with underlying rhythm
- QRS duration: As with underlying rhythm

### Clinical Significance

Identification of the mechanical impairment to cardiac output is critical in treating the patient with PEA. The longer the delay in identifying the cause the less success in correction and return to functional cardiac output. Often the causes are insurmountable, and the clinician must decide to cease resuscitation efforts.

### Proposed Interventions

1. Initiate CPR.
2. Establish airway control and IV access.
3. Initiate current advanced cardiac life support protocols such as epinephrine 1 mg every 3 to 5 minutes during arrest.
4. If PEA is associated with bradycardia, consider atropine 1 mg IV bolus, repeated every 3 to 5 minutes for a total of 3 mg.
5. Consider sodium bicarbonate depending on the patient's clinical situation.
6. Attempt to identify the cause:
   a. Confirm bilateral breath sounds (for pneumothorax).
   b. Confirm pulses with CPR (myocardial rupture, infarction, tamponade).
   c. Consider fluid challenge (hypovolemia).
   d. Assess core temperature and circumstances (hypothermia).
   e. Assess medication history (drug overdose-administer antidote).
   f. Assess blood gases (acid-base abnormality).
7. Carefully evaluate the clinical situation prior to considering cessation of efforts.

## SUMMARY

Ventricular ectopics are often signs of myocardial ischemia and hypoxia, and they frequently deteriorate into life-threatening arrhythmias. Early recognition and rapid intervention to protect the patient were the basis for the development of critical care units and paramedicine. Today automatic defibrillators are commonly available, especially in areas of mass gatherings. They are applied by laypersons, minimally trained, to an unresponsive patient. Currently advances in biotechnology have allowed for implantable cardioverters and defibrillators (ICD) to be placed without thoracatomy.

## REFERENCES

DeQuattro, V. (1998). Toward improved antihypertensive therapy with calcium-channel blockers. *Ethn Dis, 8*, 103–110.

# Chapter 9
# The AV Conduction Defects
••••••••••••••••••••••••••••••••••••••••••••••••••••••••

In the AV conduction defects (AV blocks), a pathology exists or a medication has been administered that may cause an unnatural conduction delay. AV block can be located within the AV node, infranodal, below the bundle of His, or within the bundle branches.

## BASIC GROUPING OF THE AV CONDUCTION DEFECTS

- First-degree AV block
- Second-degree AV block type I
- Second-degree AV block (a.k.a. Mobitz II)
- High or advanced second-degree AV block
- Complete AV block (a.k.a. third-degree AV block)
- Wenckebach phenomenon

## Approach to Interpretation

1. Plot out P waves, calculating rate and rhythm.
2. Plot out QRS complexes, calculating rate and rhythm.
3. Confirm the association between each P wave and the QRS complex.
4. Interpret the configuration and morphology using more than one ECG lead.
5. Determine if the rhythm is appropriate to the patient.

## First-Degree AV Block

First-degree AV block is a simple, consistent delay in conduction, usually at the level of the AV node (see Figure 9-1).

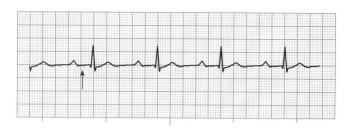

**Figure 9-1**  First-degree AV block.

### Possible Causes

- AV node ischemia (right coronary artery [RCA] disease)
- Digitalis
- Endocarditis, myocarditis, pericarditis
- Inferior wall myocardial infarction (IWMI)
- Hyperkalemia
- Lev's disease
- Lenègre's disease
- Normal variant

### ECG Characteristics

- Pacemaker site: SA node
- P waves: Single (+) P for each and every QRS complex
- PR interval: Greater than 0.20 second and consistent
- QRS complex: 0.10 second usually
  - Rate: 60 to 100/minute
  - Rhythm: Regular or slightly irregular

### Clinical Significance

First-degree AB block is usually benign in itself but in the setting of an acute infarction may lead to higher degree AV defect. Question if the patient is on or has been recently prescribed digitalis preparation.

*Proposed Interventions*

1. If the patient is asymptomatic, be supportive.
2. If symptomatic, hypotensive, and hypoperfusing, assess ABCs, $O_2$, IV, ?meds, ?med Hx, ?vital signs, ?allergies.
3. Identify cause, for example, medication such as digitalis preparation or an acute clinical condition.
4. It is rarely necessary to intervene unless bradycardia is present and the patient is symptomatic, hypotensive, and hypoperfusing.

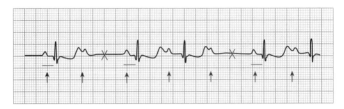

(A)

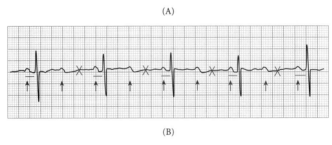

(B)

**Figure 9-2** Second-degree AV block, with an irregular (A) and regular (B) ventricular rhythm. Note the consistent PR interval after the missed QRS. In each case, sinus P waves plot through at a regular rhythm.

## Second-Degree AV Block Type I

Second-degree AV block is an intermittent conduction defect in that there is a missing QRS complex. Type I AV block usually involves AV nodal pathology, and the QRS is usually normal in duration (see Figure 9-2).

## Possible Causes

- Digitalis
- Increased parasympathetic tone
- Inferior MI
- Ischemic heart disease
- Medications
- Rarely occurs as a normal variant

### ECG Characteristics

- Pacemaker site is sinus or atrial.
- P waves: Upright, normal, (+), plot through; each QRS has a P wave to the left of it; not all P waves have a QRS following.
- PR interval: Becomes progressively longer until QRS is dropped, then the cycle is repeated. After the dropped QRS, the PR interval is the same each instance.
  a. Wenckebach phenomenon: PR interval is progressively prolonged, until there is no ventricular conduction, hence the dropped QRS.
  b. Produces a cyclic pattern of increasingly longer PR intervals until one impulse is completely blocked; cyclic pattern may be constant or variable (e.g., 2:1, 5:4, 3:2, 11:10, etc.).
- QRS complex: 0.10 second or less.
  - Rate: May be normal or slowed.
  - Rhythm: Atrial—regular unless an underlying sinus arrhythmia.

### Clinical Significance

Second-degree AV block can compromise cardiac output if it occurs in the setting of a bradycardia. Second-degree AV block is often a transient rhythm after IWMI.

### Proposed Interventions

1. If the patient is asymptomatic, be supportive.
2. If symptomatic, assess ABCs, $O_2$, IV, ?meds, ?med Hx, ?vital signs, and ?allergies.
3. Identify cause, for example, medication or an acute clinical condition.
4. Rarely necessary to intervene unless bradycardia is present and the patient is symptomatic, hypotensive, and hypoperfusing.
5. Consider preparations for transcutaneous or transvenous pacing depending on the patient's presentation.
6. Consider fluids.
7. Consider vasopressor for perfusion such as dopamine 2.5 to 10 µg/kg/minute.

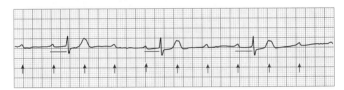

**Figure 9-3**  Advanced second-degree AV block. Note that the PR intervals are consistent; more than one QRS complex is missing and sinus P wave plot through at a regular rhythm.

## Advanced Second-Degree AV Block

High or advanced second-degree AV block is an intermittent conduction defect characterized by two or more P waves not conducted to ventricles; the ratio of conduction may be constant or variable. In either case, the PR interval after the missing (dropped) QRS is consistent (see Figure 9-3).

### Possible Causes

- Digitalis
- Inferior MI
- Ischemic heart disease
- Increased parasympathetic tone

- Medications
- Normal variant

---

### ECG Characteristics

- Pacemaker site: SA node.
- P waves: Upright, normal, (+), plot through; each QRS has a P wave to the left of it; many P waves do not have a QRS following.
- PR interval: 0.12 to 0.20 second; may be greater than 0.21 second, consistent after the missing (dropped) QRS.
- Rate: Atrial rate-unaffected; ventricular rate usually less than 60/minute.
- Rhythm: Irregular due to the missing QRS complex.

---

### Clinical Significance

In advanced second-degree AV block, the resulting bradycardia can compromise cardiac output and/or lead to complete block.

### Proposed Interventions

1. If the patient is asymptomatic, be supportive.
2. If symptomatic, assess ABCs, $O_2$, IV, ?meds, ?med Hx, ?vital signs, and ?allergies.
3. Identify cause, for example, medication or an acute clinical condition.
4. Rarely necessary to intervene unless bradycardia is present and the patient is symptomatic, hypotensive, and hypoperfusing.
5. Consider medication currently accepted for increasing the rate, such as atropine 0.5 mg IV bolus, repeated every 3 to 5 minutes (0.04 mg/kg max).
6. Consider fluids.
7. Consider vasopressor for perfusion such as dopamine 2.5 to 10 µg/kg/minute for perfusion.
8. Consider transcutaneous or transvenous pacer.

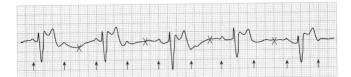

**Figure 9-4**   Second-degree AV block type II.

## Second-Degree AV Block Type II

In second degree AV block type II, the disease is at the level of or inferior to the bundle of His; therefore, the QRS complex is broader than 0.10 second. The PR interval is usually within normal limits provided there is not a coincidental AV block. Some P waves are not conducted to ventricles, and the ratio of conduction may be constant or variable (see Figure 9-4).

*Possible Causes*

- AWMI
- Septal necrosis

*ECG Characteristics*

- Pacemaker site is the sinus node.
- P waves: Upright, normal, (+), plot through; each QRS has a P wave to the left of it; many P waves do not have a QRS following. PR interval is consistent after the dropped QRS.
- QRS complex: Greater than 0.10 second, often greater than 0.12 second.
- Rate: Often associated with bradycardia.
- Rhythm: Overall irregular because of the dropped QRS. When the ventricular rhythm is regular, there is a fixed ratio of atrial to ventricular activity.

*Clinical Significance*

Second-degree AV block type II is often irreversible. Also, the resulting bradycardia can compromise cardiac output and lead to complete AV block.

### *Proposed Interventions*

1. Asymptomatic patients are rare; if so, be supportive and vigilant.
2. If the patient is symptomatic, assess ABCs, $O_2$, IV, ?meds, ?med Hx, ?vital signs, and ?allergies.
3. Identify cause, for example, medication or an acute clinical condition.
4. Set up for transcutaneous or transvenous pacemaker, because this arrhythmia is ominous.
5. Consider medication currently accepted for increasing the rate, such as atropine 0.5 mg IV bolus, repeated every 3 to 5 minutes (0.04 mg/kg max). Document the atrial rate in the interpretation of the ECG. If the atrial rate is greater than 100/minute, atropine may not be appropriate.
6. Consider fluids.
7. Consider vasopressor for perfusion such as dopamine 2.5 to 10 µg/kg/minute .

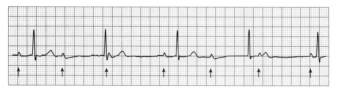

**Figure 9-5** Complete AV block, narrow QRS, probably junctional rhythm.

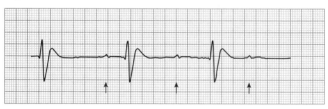

**Figure 9-6** Complete AV block, ventricular escape rhythm.

## Complete AV Block

Complete AV block exists when the atria and ventricles beat independently. Atrial depolarization is usually from the sinus

node but can be atrial flutter or fibrillation. Ventricular depolarization is from an escape junctional or ventricular mechanism (see Figures 9-5 and 9-6).

### Possible Causes

- MI
- Digitalis toxicity
- Lenègre's disease
- Lev's disease

### ECG Characteristics

- Pacemaker site: SA node and AV junction or ventricle.
- P waves: Upright, normal, (+), plot through.
- PR interval: There is no PR interval, since there is no
  AV conduction.
- QRS complex:
  a. 0.10 second if junctional in origin
  b. Greater than 0.10 second; QRS/T wave polarity if
     ventricular in origin
  - Rate: 40 to 60/minute if junctional escape; 15 to
    40/minute if ventricular escape.
  - Rhythm: Regular.

### Clinical Significance

Complete AV block can severely compromise cardiac output if
associated with AWMI or if dependent on a ventricular escape
mechanism.

### Proposed Interventions

1. Asymptomatic patients are rare; if so, be supportive and
   vigilant.
2. If the patient is symptomatic, assess ABCs, $O_2$, IV,
   ?meds, ?med Hx, ?vital signs, and ?allergies.
3. Identify cause, for example, medication or an acute clinical condition.

4. Note the atrial rate and relay that to the physician.
   a. If QRS is 0.10 second and atrial rate is 80/minute or less, consider atropine .5 mg IV bolus, repeated every 3 to 5 minutes (0.04 mg/kg max).
   b. If the QRS is greater than 0.10 second, or atrial rate is greater than 80/minute and the patient is symptomatic, hypotensive, and hypoperfusing, or if there is an idioventricular escape rhythm, set up for immediate trancutaneous or transvenous pacing.
   c. If junctional rhythm and the patient is stable, be supportive; have pacemaker on standby and the appropriate medications.
5. Consider fluids.
6. Consider vasopressor for perfusion such as dopamine 2.5 to 10 μg/kg/minute.
7. Consider transcutaneous or transvenous pacer.

## Wenckebach Phenomenon

The Wenckebach phenomenon is a progressive lengthening of conduction time in any part of cardiac tissue. It is most often associated with the AV node and is characterized by a progressive prolongation of the PR interval with the ultimate dropping of a QRS complex. The PR interval after the dropped QRS is consistently the same.

Typically, the greatest increase is between the initial and the next PR segment of the PR interval. Thereafter, as each PR segment increases, it is with decreasing increments.

The Wenckebach phenomenon can be seen with atrial fibrillation and atrial flutter, and is usually associated with digitalis toxicity. R-R intervals progressively shorten and the cycle repeats itself.

## SUMMARY

In the AV conduction defects, there is a pathology that exists or a medication has been administered that caused an unnatural conduction delay or rendered the AV node refractoy. The AV conduction defects often result in bradycardia.

Although the precise pathology of an AV conduction defect may not be immediately obvious, specific clues are visible on the ECG. It is critical to assess and evaluate the patient since blindly and reflexively attempting to accelerate the rate may further compromise the patient.

## REFERENCES

Conover, M.D., *Understanding electrocardiography: Arrhythmias and the 12-lead ECG* (7th Edition).  St Louis Mo: Mosby-Year Book, Inc.; 1998.

Marriott, H.J., & Conover, M.D.  (1998) *Advanced concepts in arhythmias*, (3rd Edition). St Louis, MO: Mosby, Inc.

# Chapter 10
# Electronic Pacemakers and Pacer Function
••••••••••••••••••••••••••••••••••••••••••••••••••••••••••••

The purpose of electronic pacing is to provide an energy source that will guarantee a minimum ventricular rate when the heart's conduction system cannot.

## COMMON FEATURES OF A PACEMAKER

1. Pacer artifact (spike) associated with the paced chamber
   a. Spike with a P wave: atrial paced complex
   b. Spike with a QRS: ventricular paced complex
   c. Spike before P and QRS in sequence: dual-chamber paced complex
2. Pacer spike plus the paced complex = electronic capture
3. Pulse with each paced ventricular complex = mechanical capture

## INDICATIONS FOR THE USE OF TRANSCUTANEOUS OR TRANSVENOUS PACING

1. Bradycardia is present and the patient is symptomatic, hypotensive, and hypoperfusing.
2. Bradycardia is present and the patient is hypotensive, hypoperfusing, and unresponsive to pharmacological intervention to accelerate the rate, for example, with atropine.
3. Bradycardia is present and the patient is asymptomatic in the presence of the following:
   a. AV block at the level of the bundle branches
   b. Characteristics of Type II AV block
   c. Complete AV block
4. SA arrest with frequent and/or prolonged episodes.
5. AWMI with evidence of the following:

   a. Right bundle branch block
   b. Left anterior fascicular block
   c. Complete left bundle branch block
6. Acute IWMI with bradycardia and the following:
   a. PVCs
   b. Complete AV block
   c. Hypotension/hypoperfusion
7. Atrial flutter or fibrillation with junctional escape rhythm.
8. Bradycardia in the setting of digitalis toxicity.
9. Induced AB block following ablation procedures.
10. Recurrent vasovagal (neurocardiogenic) syncope.
11. Long Q-T syndrome.
12. Dilated cardiomyopathy.

## PACEMAKER COMPONENTS

1. The *pulse generator* is the pacer's energy source.
   a. A transcutaneous pacemaker is external to the patient and delivers a current through the skin from one electrode to another. Transcutaneous pacemakers are manufactured separately or incorporated into defibrillator/monitors. Some are designed with a pacing cassette to be inserted into the defibrillator console, and others have pacing controls integrated into the system.
   b. The pulse generator for transvenous pacemakers can be external or implanted.
   c. *Implanted pacemakers* are encased in titanium or stainless steel housing that is hermetically sealed to protect the circuitry.
2. *Pacing electrodes* or catheters are the link between the pacemaker and the heart. A transvenous pacemaker uses a pacing catheter that is connected to the pacemaker and threaded into the right ventricle so that it contacts the right ventricular endocardium. Pacemakers deliver current through the electrodes (catheters), and in some

pacing systems, the electrodes transmit the heart's intrinsic electrical activity back to the pacemaker.

a. Transvenous pacemaker catheters are inserted using a venous approach so that the distal tip is in the right ventricle.

b. Pacemaker catheters are either bipolar or unipolar.

- Bipolar catheters have positive and negative electrodes that contact heart tissue. The distal, negative electrode is the stimulating electrode.
- Unipolar electrodes have only the negative electrode at the distal tip of the catheter. The positive or indifferent electrode is part of the pulse generator. Unipolar systems are very sensitive to intracardiac as well as extracardiac signals.

c. Noninvasive, transcutaneous pacing (TCP) electrodes are large, pregelled patches that can be anterior-posterior (AP) or anterior-left lateral (AL). The AP placement is most common and does not interfere with defibrillation, if needed (see Figure 10-1). The landmarks for placement of the TCP electrodes are well defined by the manufacturer, and the polarity should not be reversed. If the electrodes are reversed, failure to capture may occur.

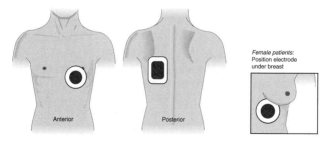

**Figure 10-1**  Example of anterior/posterior placement of transcutaneous pacemaker electrodes. Insert shows the position of the anterior electrode for patients with full, dependent breast tissue.

External pacing electrodes may be multifunctional (ECG monitoring, defibrillation/synchronized cardioversion, and pacing) or single function (pacing only). Whatever the capabilities of the electrodes, during demand pacing the patient's ECG must be monitored through ECG electrodes. Current technology does not permit multifunction electrodes to pace and monitor the patient at the same time. The repetitive pacing current is usually large compared with the intrinsic ECG and would disrupt the ECG display.

The proximity of TCP pacing electrodes to the ECG electrodes may cause artifact and distortion on the ECG. The ECG electrodes should be placed far enough away from the site of the pacemaker electrodes so that the ECG tracing is clear and distinct. For instance, the left leg electrode usually placed under the rib cage can be placed on the left side of the abdomen, away from any bony prominence or even placed on the left thigh.

## Pacemaker Energy

The current output from the pacemaker is measured in terms of milliamperes (mAs). The amount of mAs, or signal, must be of such an amplitude to cause capture but not so strong as to cause diaphragmatic pacing. The minimum amount of current required to elicit electronic and mechanical capture is called *threshold*.

*Sensitivity* is the ability of the pacemaker to process the heart's intrinsic signals and is programmed in millivolts (mVs). When the sensitivity is set at its smallest number, the pacemaker senses all intrinsic signals. As the sensitivity is set at a larger number, the pacemaker progressively ignores intrinsic signals.

For example, pacemakers set at a zero or lower are sensitive to the heart's function as with demand pacing. Conversely, if the pacemaker sensitivity is set at a large number, the pacemaker would function at a fixed-rate mode, or synchronously.

When depolarization is not sensed, the pacemaker is said to be *undersensing*. Some ectopic intrinsic activity may vary in amplitude, and the pacemaker may not be sensed by a normally operating pacemaker. When interference is sensed as if it were a depolarization wave form, the pacemaker is said to be *oversensing*. In a transcutaneous system, a higher current of output is required to overcome chest wall resistance, which is painful to an awake patient. The possibility of skin burn is minimized by the large surface area of the pregelled pacing pads.

## Pacemaker Codes

The five-letter pacemaker identification code of the Intersociety Committee on Heart Disease (ICHD) was designed to explain how a pacemaker operates and provide a consistent method of evaluating and documenting ECG characteristics of pacemakers.

The first letter of the code does not mean right and left; it indicates the chamber being paced. The second letter indicates the chamber being sensed, and the third indicates the mode of pacemaker response.

**Table 10-1** Three Letters of the Five-Letter code

| 1. Chamber paced | 2. Chamber sensed | 3. Mode of pacer response |
|---|---|---|
| V = ventricle | V = ventricle | I = inhibited |
| A = atrium | A = atrium | T = triggered |
| D = dual (both) atrium and ventricle | D = dual (both) atrium and ventricle | D = dual (both) triggered and inhibited |
| O = no chamber is paced | O = no chamber activity is sensed | O = no pacer response |

Commonly, the first three letters of the code are used to describe pacemaker activity. For example, in a demand, single-chamber (ventricular) pacer, both sensing and pacing circuits are used. Thus, this pacer would be called a VVI pacer; V= the ventricular chamber being paced, V= the intrinsic ventricular activity being sensed, and I = the ventricular function inhibited by the sensed intrinsic QRS.

Another example is the DDD pacemaker. The first D means dual-pacing activity; both atrial and ventricular chambers are paced. The second D means dual-sensing activity; both atrial and ventricular intrinsic activities are being sensed. The third D identifies what the pacer will do (pace or not) based on a sensed event.

For example, a sensed event in the atrium inhibits atrial pacing and triggers a ventricular pacing stimulus after the programmed A-V interval. A sensed beat in the ventricle inhibits the pacer's output in the ventricle.

The fourth letter stands for the type of changes or the programmability that can be made by noninvasive means:

P - programmability of rate and/or output

R - rate modulation

C - communicating

M - multiprogrammable.

These include rate, energy output, ability to sense, refractory period, and other variables as technology increases.

The fifth letter stands for the response of the pulse generator to sensing tachycardias and reflects the antitachycardia function; it varies with each manufacturer.

## CLASSIFICATION

Pacemakers are classified according to their activity, as either asynchronous or demand pacemakers.

1. Asynchronous pacemakers (VOO)
   a. Also called fixed-rate or continuous pacemakers, these generate a current at a fixed, preset rate.
   b. These pacemakers are used in congenital AV block. A fixed-rate or continuous pacemaker fires continuously regardless of the patient's intrinsic rhythm.
   c. The possibility of a pacing stimulus firing during the heart's vulnerable period is great, and the patient could suffer pacer-induced ventricular tachycardia or fibrillation.
   d. There is no sensing mechanism in a fixed-rate pacemaker.

2. Demand pacemakers (VVI/AAI)
   a. Also called ventricular-inhibited or atrial-inhibited, these pacemakers fire only when needed, that is, on demand. Demand or synchronous pacemakers have a sensing device and a timer that is preset for a specific rate, or escape interval.
   b. The sensing mechanism interprets the signal received from the patient's rhythm, allowing for intrinsic function. If an impulse is sensed within the pacemaker's preset rate, the pacemaker is inhibited, it does not pace, and the timer is reset.
   c. If an impulse is not generated after the appropriate interval, the pacer fires, and the timer is again reset. Usually the distance between the intrinsic QRS and the first paced QRS (R-V interval) is the same as the distance between two consecutive paced beats (V-V interval).
3. Rate-responsive pacemakers
   Rate-responsive, demand pacemakers are designed and programmed to respond to measurable physiological changes. These pacemakers are sensitive to the patient's activity, respiratory rate, blood temperature, metabolic status, and blood pH. Once the sensing mechanism processes the information, the pacemaker determines what the desired rate should be and increases or decreases accordingly.
4. Overdrive suppression
   a. Overly excitable myocardial tissue can result in unwelcome tachycardias that recur and may render the patient unstable, as with torsade de pointes, some atrial tachycardias, atrial flutter, PSVT, and ventricular tachycardia.
   b. In any of these situations, the application of transvenous or transcutaneous pacing at an R-V interval less than the intrinsic normal QRS-to-ectopic interval may prevent recurrence of the tachycardia until other therapies can be invoked.

c. During the temporary pacing at these high rates, the voltage and rate can be lowered slowly until a reasonable rate range is reached. If the ectopic recurs, the rate and voltage can be increased to regain control.

## THE LANGUAGE OF PACEMAKER FUNCTION

The names given to pacemaker-generated wave forms and intervals differentiate them from the patient's intrinsic wave forms and intervals.

1. *A* refers to pacer-induced atrial depolarization.
2. *Committed* is a term used in dual-chambered pacing, when ventricular stimulation occurs after atrial stimulation at a preset interval.
   a. *Fully committed* refers to ventricular stimulation that is programmed to always occur after atrial stimulation. When normal or paced atrial excitation occurs and normal (intrinsic) AV conduction results, ventricular pacing will be inhibited.
   b. *Partially committed* refers to pacemakers that have *safety pacing*. For example, after the atrial spike occurs, the pacemaker looks for any sensed event within 110 ms. If a ventricular event is sensed during that time, the pacemaker forces a ventricular spike at the end of 110 ms. If nothing is sensed during the first 110 ms after the atrial spike, the pacer will inhibit on any ventricular sensed event after 110 ms or it will pace at the end of the AV interval.
3. *V-A interval* is the time between paced ventricular and paced atrial activity.
4. *V-V interval* is the distance measured between two paced ventricular events.
5. *R-V interval* is the pacemaker's escape interval, the distance measured from the intrinsic ventricular event and the paced ventricular event that follows.
6. *Notation* is a set of numbers indicating pacer mode and programmed timing parameters, seen on the patient's

identification card. For example, a notation may be 60/160/150.

- 60 refers to the lower rate limit. The pacemaker is programmed to track spontaneous rate, and if this intrinsic rate falls below 60/minute, the pacer is programmed to provide the stimulus.
- 160, in dual-chambered pacing, refers to the A-V interval as measured in milliseconds; for example, 160 ms = 0.16 second.
- 150 refers to the pacemaker's programmed maximum rate of delivery. In this example, the paced rate should never exceed 150/minute.

7. The *escape interval* is the time from the last sensed beat to the first pacer spike. The duration of the escape interval is preset according to the desired rate.

a. For example, if the preset rate is 60/minute, the escape interval is 1 second, or five large blocks on ECG paper. A pacer-induced QRS should occur within 1 second of the previously sensed QRS complex.

b. Similarly if the preset rate is 75/minute, the escape interval is 0.8 second, or four large blocks on the ECG paper. If the patient rate drops below the preset rate, the pacemaker will guarantee the minimal preset rate. In most demand pacemakers, the escape interval is programmed to be constant.

c. If the sensing electrodes are located in the atrium, the pacemaker senses the patient's intrinsic atrial depolarization. If the sensing electrodes are located in the ventricle, the pacemaker senses the patient's intrinsic ventricular depolarization.

8. *Hysteresis* is a feature of some permanent pacemakers that allows for programming of a longer escape interval between the intrinsic complex and the first paced event. It is a delay mechanism to allow more time for the intrinsic pacemaker to generate a natural impulse. This prolonged interval should be the same every time it occurs and should occur only between the intrinsic and

first paced event. Hysteresis may easily be confused with failure to function.

**Table 10-2** Analogous Terminology for Intrinsic and Pacemaker Wave Forms and Measurements

| Intrinsic wave forms | Pacemaker term |
| --- | --- |
| P wave | A wave |
| PR interval | AV interval |
| P-P interval | A-A interval |
| QRS complex | V wave |
| R-R interval | V-V interval |
| QRS-P interval | V-A interval |
| QRS-paced QRS | R-V interval (the pacer escape interval) |

When referring to the intervals between intrinsic function and pacing function, the terminology provides an easy explanation. For example, in atrial pacing, the interval between the intrinsic P wave and the paced atrial beat is the P-A interval. Similarly, the interval between the intrinsic QRS and the paced QRS is the R-V interval (see Figure 10-2).

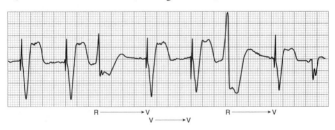

**Figure 10-2** An ECG tracing indicating R-V and V-V intervals. Note that the R-V interval is the same for narrow QRS and wide QRS ectopic complexes.

## PACEMAKER ARTIFACT AND PACER-INDUCED QRS COMPLEXES

When a pacemaker stimulus is delivered, a sharp, perfectly vertical artifact is seen on the ECG. This is called the pacer artifact, or *spike.* On the ECG, the pacemaker spike of a unipolar system usually generates a signal (the pacer spike) that is larger than the stimulus from a bipolar signal. Sometimes bipolar spikes are difficult to see. In some, the sensitivity is such that the pacer artifact may not be seen at all.

Each pacer spike will be seen on the ECG in direct association with the wave form of the chamber being paced. This association is called *electronic capture.* When a pacer spike occurs at the appropriate time and no QRS complex is associated with it, this is called *failure to capture.* Regardless of the amplitude and direction of every pacer-induced QRS, every captured QRS should result in mechanical capture, that is, a palpable carotid pulse.

## Complications and Problems with Pacemakers

1. *Failure-to-sense* describes the occurrence of premature pacing (see Figure 10-3). The pacemaker fires without regard to the patient's intrinsic function and competes with the patient for control of the heart rate. The chamber involved may respond to the pacing stimulus or not, depending on the state of refractoriness of the tissue involved. The danger here is that the pacing spike may fall during the vulnerable period of the cardiac cycle, causing repetitive firing, ventricular tachycardia, or fibrillation.

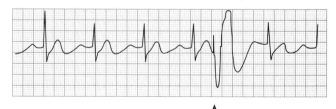

**Figure 10-3** An ECG tracing showing failure to sense. Note the paced complex (arrow) is premature and dangerously close to the previous T wave.

2. Failure-to-capture is when
   a. a pacer spike fails to produce the paced complex (see Figure 10-4) **or**
   b. the pacer-induced QRS fails to produce a pulse.
   Failure-to-capture may be a problem with the position of the catheter or inadequate voltage. Failure-to-capture may also reflect the inability of the heart to respond to the stimulus.

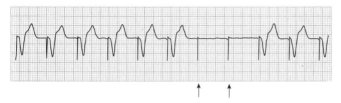

**Figure 10-4** An ECG tracing of a ventricular paced rhythm with two episodes of failure to capture (arrows).

3. *Dislodgement* of the transvenous catheter can result in failure-to-capture or inappropriate stimulation. If the position of the catheter changes, the paced ECG pattern will change. One complication is perforation of the ventricular septum (see Figure 10-5). In this instance, the catheter electrode may penetrate the ventricular septum and "pace" from the left ventricle. Although the pacer stimulus (spike) may be seen on the ECG, there may not be a captured QRS complex. An indication of perforate septum is a positive pacer-induced QRS.

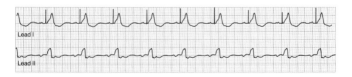

**Figure 10-5** An example of positive (+) paced QRS complexes in a patient with documented perforated septum.

4. *Endocardial puncture* is when the catheter perforates the myocardium. The paced QRS will be positive. Endocardial puncture may result in myocardial tamponade.
5. *Pacer-induced tachycardia* occurs in dual-chambered pacing. If there is retrograde conduction from the ventricular beat and the retrograde P wave is sensed by the pacemaker *after* the atrial and the ventricular pacemaker refractory periods, a tachycardia will develop. The pacemaker will have to be reprogrammed to extend the atrial refractory period or switch to a DVI mode of pacing, thereby eliminating sensing atrial activity.
6. *Interference* is when the pacemaker senses a type and amplitude of an external source of energy and is unable to discriminate between intrinsic electrical forces and the unknown source. For example, the pacer will be inhibited from functioning when near a microwave or certain cellular telephones, digital, analog, and 900 MHz cordless phones. This would endanger the patient, especially if the patient is totally dependent on the pacer and it will not fire. A safe working distance is recommended for those using these devices.
7. Equipment breakage.
8. Infection—anywhere along the path of the wire.
9. Pacemaker Syndrome.
   a. Usually due to inadequate pacer rate
   b. This leads to low cardiac output, particularly during exertion
   c. Result may be heart failure, with fatigue, shortness of breath, and chest pain
   d. Most common in patients with VVI pacers and sinus (SA) node dysfunction

### Proposed Interventions

1. TCP is implemented in cases of bradycardia in a patient who is hypotensive and hypoperfusing.
2. TCP is also indicated in patients with MI where bundle branch block is present.

3. TCP is maintained for a very short period of time, usually minutes or less than 1 hour.
4. Transvenous pacing is indicated for similar clinical problems and can be maintained for a few days.
5. Patients with implanted pacemakers with identified problems such as failure-to-function, failure-to-sense, and failure-to-capture can benefit by application of TCP.
6. Patients with implanted pacemakers with ventricular tachycardia or fibrillation can be defibrillated. The defibrillator electrodes must be at least 5 inches away from the pacemaker.
7. Patients with PVCs can be treated with lidocaine, because in therapeutic doses, lidocaine will not affect the myocardial response to pacemaker energy.

To assess pacemaker function, approach the ECG step by step:

1. Whenever possible, identify the patient's underlying rhythm.
2. Identify the mode of pacing: demand versus asynchronous.
3. Evaluate the pacer: To identify a pacer in the demand mode, you must see the patient's own intrinsic QRS.
   a. Measure the distance between two paced beats (the pacing interval).
   b. Compare the distance between the patient's last normal beat and the first paced beat (the escape interval, sometimes called the demand interval). These measurements should be the same (i.e., the paced interval equals the escape interval). The documentation will include identification of the patient's rhythm and rate and an assessment of the pace: for example, "atrial fib at 70 to 85 beats/minute, a ventricular demand pacer at 72 beats/minute. The escape and paced intervals are constant." Recall that the demand pacer is set or timed to function within the escape interval. That interval should not change. If meas-

urements reveal that the R-V interval is longer or shorter than what is expected, this is reportable, because the pacer may not be functioning properly (see Figure 10-6).

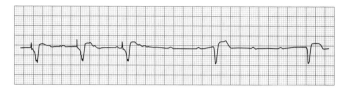

**Figure 10-6**  ECG showing failure to function.

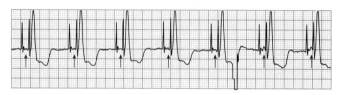

**Figure 10-7**  An ECG tracing of a dual-chamber pacemaker. Note the fixed A-V intervals.

## ASSESSING A DUAL-CHAMBER PACEMAKER ON THE ECG

1. Identify the patient's underlying rhythm.
2. Evaluate the escape interval.
   a. Measure the distance between the first of the pacer artifacts for two paced beats.
   b. Plot back in time and determine which wave forms match this interval, that is, the patient's P wave or the QRS complex. This will indicate which complex is being sensed by the pacer.
3. Measure the AV interval, its value, and its consistency (see Figure 10-7).
4. Assess the patient's pulse and perfusion. Assess for dizziness, episodes of fainting, edema, dyspnea, chest pain, and hiccough.

## Clinical Implications

The dual-chambered pacer is programmed to provide both atrial and ventricular function in sequence, to provide as near normal perfusion as possible. It is important to determine how the pacer functions in terms of its sensing capabilities as well as the patient's pulse and perfusion. Assess for dizziness, episodes of fainting, edema, dyspnea, chest pain, and hiccough.

## SUMMARY

The function of the electronic pacemaker is to provide an artificial stimulus when the heart's own electrical system fails. Advancing technology has increased pacemaker options for a variety of problems. With the increase in variability of application comes an increase in complexity.

The function of all pacemakers should be assessed to determine problems with failure to function, sense, and capture. A consistent approach to ECG rhythm analysis will help the clinician detect problems with any of these functions and assess the patient's physical and mental well-being.

## REFERENCES

Trigano AJ; Azoulay A; Rochdi M; Campillo A. (1999). Electromagnetic interference of external pacemakers by walkie-talkies and digital cellular phones: experimental study. *Pacing Clin Electrophysiol 22,* 588-93.

# Chapter 11
# Arrhythmias Due to Abnormal Conduction Pathways
••••••••••••••••••••••••••••••••••••••••••••••••••••••

A wide QRS does not always imply PVCs, ventricular tachycardia, or bundle branch block. An accessory pathway is an extra muscle bundle that exists outside the normal, specialized conduction tissue, sometimes termed "bypass tracts," as they bypass the AV node. This bundle forms a connection between the atria and ventricles, allowing for early activation of the ventricles, hence preexcitation. *Preexcitation syndrome* is used to describe clinical situations where preexcitation causes tachycardias.

## CLINICAL IMPLICATIONS

Preexcitation is of concern because there is a potential for supraventricular tachyarrhythmias to occur.

1. PSVT and atrial fibrillation that result from an unrecognized preexcitation syndrome can deteriorate into ventricular fibrillation. In some cases of preexcitation, the resulting QRS complex is widened and may be confused with bundle branch block.
2. Wide QRS complex arrhythmias occurring with preexcitation may be confused with ventricular tachycardia.

## PHYSIOLOGY OF THE ACCESSORY PATHWAY (AP)

1. *Kent bundles* are accessory AV pathways that connect the atrium to the ventricles, outside the normal conduction system (see Figure 11-1A).
2. The James bundle is an accessory pathway that connects atrial fibers to the upper part of the AV node. This is also termed an *intranodal bypass tract* (see Figure 11-1B).

3. Mahaim's fibers are accessory pathways that connect the AV node and the ventricle (*nodoventricular*), the bundle of His and the bundle branch (*nodofascicular*), or the bundle branch and the ventricles (*fascicular ventricular*) (see Figure 11-1C).

4. *Atriofascicular bypass tracts* are fibers that connect the atrium to the bundle of His.

5. Concealed accessory pathway is an accessory pathway that conducts only in a retrograde direction. During sinus rhythm, conduction down the AV junction, through to and within the ventricles, is normal. The PR interval and QRS duration are within normal limits, and there is no delta wave.

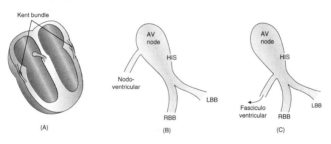

**Figure 11-1** (A) The site of the Kent bundles, (B) the James bundle, and (C) Mahaim's fibers. (Adapted from Conover, M.B. *Understanding Electrocardiography: Arrhythmias and the 12–lead ECG* (7th ed.). St. Louis, MO: Mosby-Year Book, Inc.; 1998.)

## Possible Causes

Causes of preexcitation are usually congential.

### ECG Wave Forms Affected by Preexcitation

- The ECG pattern of preexcitation consists primarily of a short PR interval, with the QRS narrow or wide;

*continues*

*continued*

a very rapid, irregular, and abnormally wide QRS complex, when atrial fibrillation occurs with an accessory pathway; and a *delta wave*, which is a slurring of the initial wave form of the QRS complex.

a. The polarity of the delta wave may not be seen in all leads or may not be seen at all.

b. If the forces of excitation are toward the positive electrode in a lead, the polarity of the delta wave will be positive.

c. If the forces of excitation are away from the positive electrode in a lead, the polarity of the delta wave will be negative, and it will produce an abnormal Q wave in leads III and $V_1$.

d. If the forces of excitation are perpendicular to the positive electrode in a lead, the polarity will be isoelectric and may not be visible at all.

• The amplitude of the delta wave depends on how quickly the accessory pathway conducts the current ahead of the normal wave of depolarization (see Figure 11-2).

a. If normal and accessory wave fronts arrive simultaneously, then there may be no delta wave, and the PR interval would be unchanged.

*continues*

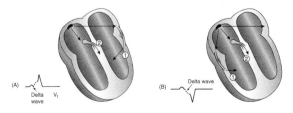

**Figure 11-2**   Graphic illustration of accessory pathway and resulting delta waves. (Adapted from Conover, M.B. *Understanding Electrocardiography: Arrhythmias and the 12–lead ECG* (7th ed.). St. Louis, MO: Mosby-Year Book, Inc.; 1998.)

*continued*

    b. Since there will be sources depolarizing the ventricles, the resulting QRS will be a fusion of both wave fronts.

- The width of the QRS depends on the following:
    a. The length of time it takes to conduct through the accessory pathway
    b. The location of the accessory pathway
    c. The accessory pathway's conduction time between the sinus and AV nodes

## DEGREES OF PREEXCITATION

About 25% of bypass tracts are capable of only retrograde conduction.

1. *None.* The patient has a latent accessory pathway, and the PR interval and QRS duration are normal (see Figure 11-3A). The anatomical source of the pathway is on the lateral side of the left ventricle. This pathway may become active with atrial fibrillation and is capable of antegrade conduction, consequently resulting in a life-threatening arrhythmia.

2. *Minimal.* The size of the delta wave is very small, and it is not seen in all leads (see Figure 11-3B).

3. *Less than maximum.* The impulse arrives in the ventricle, first using the accessory pathway (short PR interval) and then using the AV node, causing a fusion beat (see Figure 11-3C).
    a. The resulting QRS may not have the classic delta wave but may exhibit an abnormal Q wave or distortion of the ascending arm of the R wave or increased QRS voltage.
    b. In less than maximum preexcitation, it is difficult to differentiate between ventricular hypertrophy, bundle branch block, and AMI.

4. *Maximum preexcitation.* Both ventricles are activated by the accessory pathway. There is almost no PR interval, and the fusing of P to the QRS complex results in the widened QRS (see Figure 11-3D).

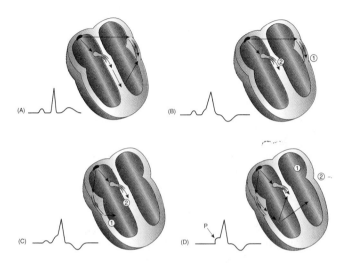

**Figure 11-3** Graphic illustration of accessory pathway and resulting delta waves with varying degrees of preexcitation: (A) normal, (B) minimal, (C) less than maximum, and (D) maximum activation. (Adapted from Conover, M.B. *Understanding Electrocardiography: Arrhythmias and the 12–lead ECG* (7th Ed.). St. Louis, MO: Mosby-Year Book, Inc.; 1998.)

## ARRHYTHMIAS ORIGINATING IN ACCESSORY PATHWAYS

- Reciprocating tachycardia
- Orthodromic tachycardia
- Antidromic tachycardia
- Lown Ganong Levine syndrome
- WPW syndrome

## Approach to Interpretation

When preexcitation is suspected, the clinician must perform the following:

1. Assess the PR interval. Recall, the PR may not be obviously shortened.
2. Look for a delta wave in all leads. Recall that a delta wave may not be visible in all leads taken simultaneously.
3. Obtain a 12-lead ECG. This must be taken during the tachycardia episode.
4. Compare the ECG with the resting or normal ECG to rule out preexcitation.

### ECG Characteristics

- P waves: P′ may be (−) or (+) in lead I and may be seen after the QRS complex.
- P′-R interval: Less than 0.12 second and constant.
- QRS complex: 0.10 second in duration. *QRS alternans* may be seen, which is alteration of the amplitude of the R and S waves of the QRS complex.
    - Rate: 60 to 100/minute.
    - Rhythm: Regular.

## Reciprocating Tachycardia

*Reciprocating tachycardia* occurs when a premature atrial focus conducts down the normal AV conduction system but uses the accessory pathway to reenter the atria. This is also called *circus-movement tachycardia*, or *reentry tachycardia*, or *orthodromic (narrow QRS) reciprocating tachycardia*.

A PVC can cause a tachycardia by entering the atria via the accessory pathway and subsequently traveling down the AV node, down the His bundle, and into the ventricles. This will result in a narrow QRS tachycardia.

During sinus tachycardia, when a critical rate is reached, the accessory pathway is blocked in an antegrade fashion. The impulse may well conduct normally and reenter the atria using the accessory pathway in a retrograde fashion, thus establishing the reentry circuit.

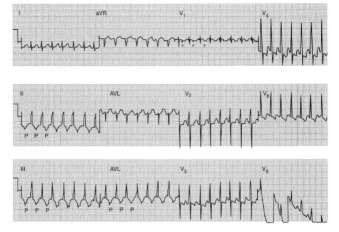

**Figure 11-4**   A 12-lead ECG showing orthodromic reciprocating tachycardia. (Adapted from Conover, M.B. *Understanding Electrocardiography: Arrhythmias and the 12–lead ECG* (7th Ed.). St. Louis, MO: Mosby-Year Book, Inc.; 1998.)

## Orthodromic Tachycardia

*Orthodromic tachycardia* can occur using a slower conducting accessory pathway (see Figure 11-4). The reentry circuit uses the AV node in an antegrade direction and a slower conducting accessory pathway in the retrograde direction. The slower conduction time from ventricle to atria over the slow accessory pathway will produce a long RP interval. In fact, the P′ will be closer to the QRS that follows it rather than the one that precedes it. At first glance, the rhythm appears as a junctional tachycardia, but the ventricular rate is much faster at 130 to 200/minute.

## Antidromic Tachycardia

*Antidromic (wide QRS) tachycardia* is a reentry tachycardia that uses the accessory pathway in an antegrade fashion and the AV node in a retrograde direction (see Figure 11-5). The resulting QRS will be wide and the ventricular rhythm may be irregular, because retrograde conduction though the ventricular pathways may differ. In some cases, a P′ will result because of the retrograde stimulation of the atria. This P′ may be seen after the QRS but not in all leads, because the QRS is so broad.

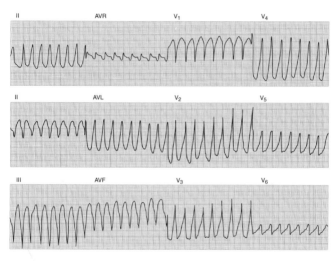

**Figure 11-5**   A 12-lead ECG showing antidromic reciprocating tachycardia. (Adapted from Conover, M.B. *Understanding Electrocardiography: Arrhythmias and the 12–lead ECG* (7th Ed.). St. Louis, MO: Mosby-Year Book, Inc.; 1998.)

The tachycardia can be caused by the use of two accessory pathways.

1. There can be antegrade conduction down one accessory pathway and retrograde conduction using another accessory pathway. In this instance the QRS will be wide

and very difficult to differentiate from ventricular tachycardia.

2. There can be atrial fibrillation conducting to the ventricles over an accessory pathway in an antegrade fashion (see Figure 11-6). This results in a ventricular rate sometimes greater than 200 beats/minute but with the irregularity that is characteristic of the atrial fibrillation.

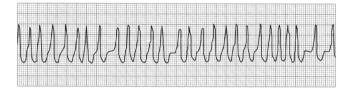

**Figure 11-6**  Lead II ECG tracing showing atrial fibrillation using an accessory pathway from a patient with diagnosed digitalis toxicity. Closely inspect the broad QRS complex, which has some (+) delta waves. (Adapted from Conover, M.B. *Understanding Electrocardiography: Arrhythmias and the 12–lead ECG* (7th Ed.). St. Louis, MO: Mosby-Year Book, Inc.; 1998.)

Conduction through a rapidly conducting accessory pathway can result in irregular ventricular activity that rapidly deteriorates into ventricular fibrillation.

## Lown Ganong Levine Syndrome

Lown Ganong Levine syndrome (LGL), also known as intranodal bypass tract syndrome, was initially described as a combination of a short PR interval, normal QRS configuration, and recurrent supraventricular tachycardia (see Figure 11-7). It was subsequently shown that in patients who exhibit LGL, intranodal fibers bypass the crest of the AV node, and one of the intranodal fibers terminates near the bundle of His (James fibers). The normal conduction delay in the AV node is thus circumvented, and a short PR interval is recorded of less than 0.12 second. Ventricular depolarization will take place via the

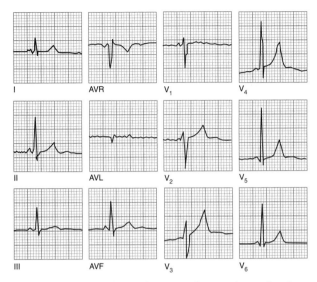

**Figure 11-7**   A 12-lead ECG showing a short PR interval and a narrow QRS complex in a patient with confirmed Lown Ganong Levine syndrome.

normal His-Purkinje system, thus generating a normal QRS complex.

---

*ECG Characteristics*
- P wave: Upright, positive in all leads
- PR interval: 0.12 second
- QRS Complex: Normal
  - Rate: Rapid, but no clinical history of tachycardia
  - Rhythm: Regular unless in the case of atrial fibrillation

Such ECG tracings probably indicate bypass of the AV node by an intranodal fiber and should be interpreted as consistent with, but not diagnostic of, the LGL presentation.

In summary, the three criteria for diagnosis of the LGL syndrome are as follows:

1. Short PR interval (0.12 second or less)
2. Normal QRS configuration
3. Recurrent paroxysmal tachycardia

## Wolff Parkinson White Syndrome

Wolff Parkinson White (WPW) is a syndrome of preexcitation that occurs using accessory AV pathways (Kent bundles) accompanied by tachycardia (see Figure 11-8). When WPW occurs without tachycardia, it is termed *WPW pattern*. WPW can occur in healthy hearts. The anatomical presence of the accessory pathway may not manifest itself until later in life or only in the presence of MI or atrial fibrillation.

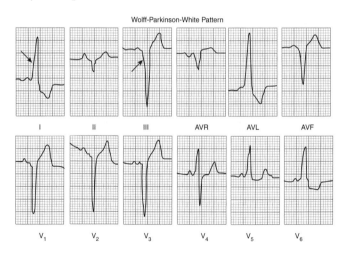

Wolff-Parkinson-White Pattern

I   II   III   AVR   AVL   AVF

V₁   V₂   V₃   V₄   V₅   V₆

**Figure 11-8**  A 12-lead ECG showing Wolff Parkinson White pattern. Delta waves (arrows) can be (+) or (−).

In WPW, as atrial tissue is depolarized and forms the P wave on ECG, the depolarizing wave front arrives simultaneously at the crest of the AV node at the atrial end of the accessory pathway.

Conduction through the AV node is normally delayed, but the accessory pathway is capable of very rapid depolarization. Thus, ventricular tissue is depolarized before the AV node has permitted normal conduction to continue through the His bundle.

If all ventricular tissue were depolarized by the impulse using the accessory pathway, the resulting QRS would be different than the sinus-induced QRS. The resulting widened QRS complexes can be confused with bundle branch block or PVCs. However, as the wave of depolarization slowly spreads out from the prematurely depolarized ventricle, conduction is completed through the AV junction and spreads quickly through the His-Purkinje system.

The net result of all of this is a composite of both initial, premature ventricular depolarization (accessory pathway) and later activation of the remaining myocardium using the normal conduction system. The initial aberrant activation generates a slurring of the QRS called the delta wave, previously explained.

The changes that occur with MI, bundle branch block, and ventricular hypertrophy will be masked by the WPW pattern. Confident, definitive diagnosis for the existence of an accessory pathway can only be made by using electrophysiological testing. Any conclusion about the electrical conduction system based on simply assessing the QRS must be discouraged.

The major clinical manifestation of WPW is recurrent tachycardia. As with LGL syndrome, the accessory pathway supports the circulating, reentrant wave of depolarization. However, unlike LGL, in WPW the resulting QRS may be normal or widened depending on the direction of the reentrant wave front.

If the AV node is activated in an antegrade fashion and the bundle of Kent is activated in a retrograde fashion, the QRS complex will be narrow. However if Kent bundle is depolarized in an antegrade fashion, with retrograde depolarization of the AV node, a wide, bizarre QRS complex will be recorded. This may mimic ventricular tachycardia. Impulses travel down the AV junction and up the bypass tract in 90% of WPW tachycardias. In 10% of the tachycardias, there is a wide-complex QRS with delta waves. Recall, delta wave may **not** be visible in all ECG leads.

---

### ECG Characteristics of Overt WPW

- P waves: Upright, normal, and appearing only before each QRS
- P-R interval: Less than 0.12 second and constant
- QRS complex: Greater than 0.10 second in duration; a delta wave, slurred on the initial upstroke or downstroke of the QRS
  - Rate: 60 to 100/minute
  - Rhythm: Regular

---

### ECG Characteristics of Nonevident WPW

- P waves: Upright, normal, and appearing only before each QRS
- P-R interval: 0.12 to 0.20 second and constant
- QRS complex: 0.10 second in duration
  - Rate: 60 to 100/minute; tendency for unprovoked PSVT, atrial flutter, or atrial fibrillation
  - Rhythm: Regular

---

### ECG Characteristics of Concealed WPW

- P waves: Upright, normal, and appearing only before each QRS
- P-R interval: 0.12 to 0.20 second and constant
- QRS complex: 0.10 second in duration
  - Rate: 60 to 100/minute; tendency for unprovoked PSVT
  - Rhythm: Regular

### Clinical Significance

Without episodes of arrhythmias, such as atrial fibrillation with rapid ventricular response or a reentrant tachycardia, an accessory pathway may not be discovered. The following should alert the clinician to the possibility of accessory pathways. If the PSVT converts with conventional intervention, the presence of the accessory pathway may not be evident since the PR interval and QRS duration will be normal. Assessment should include the following:

1. Assess leads I, II, III, $V_1$, and $V_6$ while the patient is in PSVT. The P′ wave may be seen on one lead and not others.
   a. Whenever possible, compare this tachycardia with the patient's previous sinus rhythm. With circus movement tachycardia, the P′ wave will be separate from the QRS and closer to the preceding R wave.
2. Assess heart rates. With aberrant ventricular conduction, rates are slower than without the aberrancy when the accessory pathway is on the same anatomical side as the aberrant ventricular conduction.
3. Assess ventricular rate. Ventricular rates are very rapid with sudden, unprovoked PSVT or atrial fibrillation with rapid conduction using the accessory pathway.
4. Assess ventricular rhythm. Ventricular rhythm is very irregular in the case of atrial fibrillation.
5. Assess for history of onset. A few patients with WPW will present with ventricular fibrillation without any warning.

### Proposed Interventions

1. AV nodal blocking agents should be avoided in preexcitation syndromes.
2. Medications such as
   a. Amiodarone may be especially helpful in termination of AV reciprocating tachycardia
   b. Magnesium IV may be helpful in reversing digitalis induced tachycardia

3. Patients whose paroxysms of tachycardia persist should be clinically assessed and undergo electrophysiological testing for the possibility of an active accessory pathway.

4. Surgery or transvenous radio frequency catheter ablation is the preferred modality for treating patients who become intolerant of the arrhythmias or have a predilection toward atrial fibrillation.

Table 11-1 summarizes ECG wave forms and characteristics in early excitation using accessory AV bundle, intra-AV nodal bypass tract, and nodofascicular connection.

**Table 11-1** Wave Forms and Characteristics in Early Excitation

| ECG | Accessory AV bundle | Intranodal bypass tract | Nodofascicular connection |
|---|---|---|---|
| PR Interval | <0.12 second | <0.12 second | Normal |
| QRS duration | >0.11 second | Normal* | >0.11 second |
| Secondary ST-T abnormalities | Present | Absent | Present |
| Delta Waves | Present | Absent | Present |
| Can mimic MI | Yes | No* | Yes |
| Can mimic ventricular hypertrophy | Yes | No* | Yes |

* Must rule out prior pathology in the bundle branch system.

## SUMMARY

Frequent occurrence of tachycardia without any overt cardiac disease, especially in the younger patient, may be the first sign of activation of an accessory pathway. Sometimes unexplained tachycardia is the only reported sign that heralds pathology using an abnormal conduction pathway.

### REFERENCES

Conover, M.D., *Understanding electrocardiography: Arrhythmias and the 12-lead ECG* (7th Edition). St Louis Mo: Mosby-Year Book, Inc.; 1998.

Crippa, G., Sverzellati, E., Giorgi-Pierfranceschi, M., & Carrara, G.C. (1999). Magnesium and cardiovascular drugs: interactions and therapeutic role. *Ann Ital Med Int, 14*, 40–45.

Kuga, K., Yamaguchi, I., & Sugishita, Y. (1999). Effect of intravenous amiodarone on electrophysiologic variables and on the modes of termination of antrioventricular reciprocating tachycardia in Wolff Parkinson White syndrome. *Jpn Circ, 63*, 189–195.

Marriott, H.J., & Conover, M.B. (1998) *Advanced concepts in arrhythmias*, (3rd Edition). St Louis, MO: Mosby, Inc.

Merrill, J.J., DeWeese, G., and Wharton, J.M. (1999). Magnesium reversal of digoxin-facilitated ventricular rate during atrial fibrillation in the Wolff Parkinson White syndrome. *American Journal of Medicine, 97*, 25.

# Chapter 12
# Myocardial Infarction
••••••••••••••••••••••••••••••••••••••••••••••••••••••

MI evolves through three stages: ischemia, injury, and necrosis. These debilitating processes are reflected by changes in the ECG leads that explore the affected surface of the heart. Over 80% of patients with MI have ECG changes consistent with ischemia. It is noted that a new ST Segment elevation increased likelihood of MI 5–54X and that a new Q wave increased likelihood of MI by 5–25 fold. A normal ECG reduces likelihood of MI 3–10 fold. Overall sensitivity of ECG for all MIs is 50 to 70%. The process of myocardial injury is time dependent; reperfusion increases as time-to-treatment decreases. With early recognition and reperfusion, ischemia and injury can be reversed and infarction prevented. Early recognition and rapid intervention can reduce mortality and promote left ventricular function.

## PROBABLE CAUSES

- Accumulation of atheromatous plaque
- Amphetamines
- Cocaine
- Coronary artery spasm
- Fixed atherosclerotic obstruction
- Obstructive thrombus
- Trauma

Any of the preceding situations can cause ischemia, which is a lack of perfusion of oxygenated blood. Any degree of ischemia causes cellular changes. Ischemic and injured tissue may not be able to contract appropriately, but it is still salvageable. If occlusion persists, cell death leads to necrosis, or MI, and the loss of depolarizing cardiac muscle. Prolonged QRS duration in AWMI is associated with 1.5 times increased mortality. Bundle Branch Block (BBB) may occur with the evolving MI.

With a delay in depolarization in ischemic tissue, repolarization is also delayed. This causes deep T wave inversion in the leads reflecting the affected area.

ST segment changes along with the appearance of Q waves signal an evolving MI. This is because the tissue immediately adjacent to the infarcted tissue may not be functional. Although collateral circulation may be enough to sustain cell life, perfusion is not sufficient to maintain cellular integrity. There will be a difference in electrical potential in the injured tissue, and a *current of injury* pattern will occur during repolarization, seen as ST segment elevation in the leads facing (reflecting) the injured tissue. ST segment depression is seen in a lead opposite or reciprocal to the injured area. Absolute ST deviation (depression or elevation) is associated with 1.5 times increased mortality.

MI can be transmural, or also called full thickness, or nontransmural, confined to the subendocardium. With AMI, abnormal Q waves are seen in the leads directly over (reflecting) the infarcted tissue. This results from the loss of electrical potential with cell death. The more leads in which Q waves are seen, the greater the infarct size. Q waves persist well after the event.

## REFLECTING AND RECIPROCAL LEADS

ECG signs of ischemia, injury, and necrosis are best seen in the leads facing the affected surface of the heart. These leads are called the *reflecting leads*. *Reciprocal leads* are in the same plane but opposite the event, and the ECG sign is seen as a mirror image. Recall the posterior surface is evaluated using $V_2$, $V_3$, and $V_4$ which are reciprocal (Chapter 2, Figure 2-5). Table 12-1 summarizes the reflecting leads.

Lead $V_{4R}$ is a very informative lead. ST elevation in $V_{4R}$ is 90% predictive of right ventricular wall MI. $V_{4R}$ also will help the clinician to identify three things:

- The site of coronary occlusion
  a. ST elevation and positive T waves indicate proximal occlusion of the RCA.

**Table 12-1** Reflecting Leads

| Surface of the Heart | Reflecting Leads |
| --- | --- |
| Inferior | II, III and aVF |
| Right ventricular | $V_{4R}$ |
| Posterior | Evolving: $V_1$<br>Acute: $V_2$, $V_3$, $V_4$ |
| Anterior | $V_3$ and $V_4$ |
| Extensive anterior | I, aVL and $V_3$ to $V_6$ |
| Anteroseptal | $V_1$ to $V_4$ |
| Anterolateral | I, aVL, $V_3$ to $V_6$ |
| Inferolateral | II, III and aVF (inferior)<br>I, aVL, $V_5$, $V_6$ (lateral) |
| High lateral | I and aVL |

     b. Normal ST segments and positive T waves may indicate distal RCA occlusion.

     c. Normal ST segment and negative T waves may implicate the occlusion of the circumflex artery.

- Patients at risk for AV conduction defects
- Patients who would benefit most by aggressive reperfusion techniques

In a normal heart, $V_{4R}$ through $V_{6R}$ will resemble the ECG complexes seen in lead $V_1$ but will be lower in amplitude. The posterior leads will resemble $V_6$ but also will be of lower amplitude. As in the other leads, the process of ischemia to infarction is represented by ST segment elevation, T wave inversion, or the presence of Q waves in the leads facing the affected surface of the heart. Remember, posterior infarction accompanies inferior wall MI in perhaps 30% of patients. Right ventricular involvement may occur in as many as 40% of inferior wall MI.

Finally, although the posterior surface is reflected by leads $V_7$ and $V_8$, the reciprocal leads are $V_1$–$V_4$. Figure 12-1 illustrates the surfaces of the heart, the reflecting leads, and the reciprocal leads.

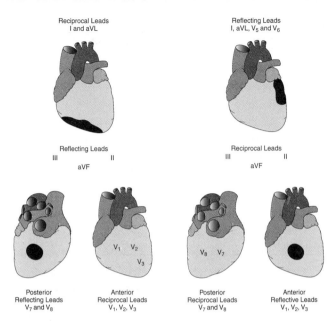

**Figure 12-1** View of the heart's surface from the reflecting and reciprocal leads.

## ST Segment Changes

Segment depression may be characterized by the following:

1. Nonspecific
2. Indicative of subendocardial (non-Q wave) infarction
3. A reciprocal change in leads opposite the area of acute injury
4. Seen during anginal attacks or during a positive stress test
5. Produced by the effects of antiarrhythmic medications, such as digitalis and quinidine
6. Produced by hypothermia
7. Seen with electrolyte imbalances such as hyperkalemia or hypokalemia
8. A normal variant in up to 20% of otherwise healthy women

ST segment elevation (J point elevation) is known as the *current of injury pattern*.

1. ST elevation greater than 1 mm in the limb leads and greater than 2 mm in the precordial leads indicates an evolving AMI till proven otherwise.
2. ST segment elevation may also be a normal variant.
3. ST segment elevation, which usually indicates that transmural injury is occurring, must be readily recognized so that reperfusion can be implemented as soon as possible.
4. The ST segment elevation associated with evolving infarction usually encompasses the T wave in its contour.
5. *Early repolarization* is a normal variant of the ST segment seen in 1% to 2% of younger, male patients.
6. Elevated, concave, ST segments are commonly located in the precordial leads.
7. ST elevation is marked by a flat or concave ST segment and usually is accompanied by T wave elevation; depressed PR segments may indicate pericarditis.
8. ST segment elevation that does not return to baseline over time may indicate ventricular aneurysm.

### Clinical Significance

The clinician must be vigilant and must maintain a high degree of suspicion for any patient who presents with chest pain of any description.

ST segment elevations related to myocardial injury usually appear convex or curved. Sometimes this is referred to as a *positive ST segment coving*. After AMI, or when ischemia has resolved, the ST segment usually returns toward baseline; this usually occurs in the first 72 to 96 hours after damage. Figure 12-2 is an ECG tracing from a patient who presented with substernal chest pain radiating to the left arm, shortness of breath, pallor, and diaphoresis; the tracing shows the changes in ST segments from time of the initial encounter to 14 minutes after oxygen therapy and nitroglycerin.

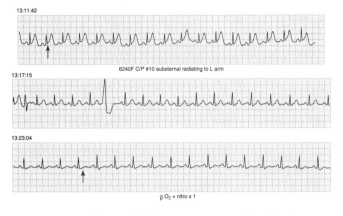

**Figure 12-2**  Inferior wall changes; response to nitroglycerin.

## Summary of the Criteria for the Diagnosis of Transmural Injury

1. Elevation of the origin of the ST segment, at 0.04 second past the J point, of 1 mm or more in two or more limb leads or precordial leads $V_4$ to $V_6$, or 2 mm or more in two or more precordial leads $V_1$ to $V_3$.
2. Depression of the origin of the ST segment at the J point 1 mm or more in two or more leads $V_1$ to $V_3$, with ST segment elevation greater than 1 mm in two or more leads $V_7$ to $V_9$.

### Minor ST Segment Depression

Minor ST segment depression may have significance in the total clinical presentation with other ECG findings. Criteria for minor ST segment depression are either of the following:

1. ST-J depression as much as 0.5 mm. ST segment downward sloping and segment or T-wave nadir at least 0.5 mm below P-R baseline, in any of leads I, II, aVL, or $V_2$ to $V_6$.

2. ST-J depression of 1.0 mm or greater and ST segment upward sloping or U-shaped, in any of leads I, II, aVL, or $V_1$ to $V_6$.

## T Wave Changes

Although the normal amplitude for T wave excursion has never been firmly established, T wave contour is susceptible to many factors:

1. T wave inversion or flattening may be a normal variant.
2. Deep, symmetrical T wave inversion suggests a diagnosis of ischemia.
3. T wave contour may be affected by exercise, food ingestion, hyperventilation, and smoking.
4. Precordial T waves that are greater than 10 mm in deflection strongly suggest hyperkalemia.
5. T waves greater than 10 mm in the right precordial leads are seen in patients with left ventricular hypertrophy.
6. Symmetrical T wave inversion in a lead that normally has an upright T wave may be clinically associated with ischemia.
7. T waves that are very symmetrical and greater than 5 mm in depth are called *nadir T waves* (see Figure 12-3).
8. Bundle branch block.
9. Ventricular hypertrophy.
10. Pericarditis.
11. Electrolyte disorders.
12. Shock.
13. Positional changes such as posturing with dyspnea, or the patient seated in an upright rather than supine position.
14. Central nervous system disorders such as subarachnoid hemorrhage and stroke.

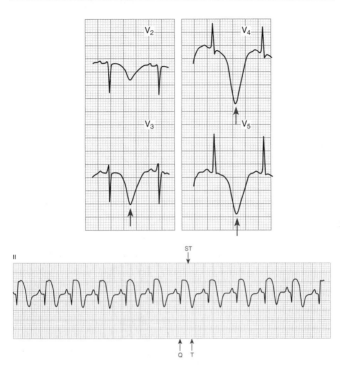

**Figure 12-3**  Nadir T waves.

## Minor T Wave Abnormalities

Minor T wave abnormalities are associated with occult cardiac events. They commonly accompany other minor wave abnormalities such as ST segment depression or elevation. Accepted criteria for minor T wave abnormalities are either of the following:

1. T wave amplitude zero (flat), negative, or diphasic (negative-positive type only) with less than 1.0 mm negative phase in leads I, II, and $V_3$ to $V_6$, or in lead aVL when R wave amplitude is 5.0 mm or greater.
2. T wave amplitude positive and T to R wave amplitude ratio of less than 1:20 in any leads I, II, aVL, or $V_3$ to $V_6$

when R wave amplitude in the corresponding leads is
10.0 mm or greater.

## Abnormal U Waves

An abnormal U wave is a frequent mark of ischemic heart disease. It is most often recorded in lead I, lead II, and precordial leads $V_5$–$V_6$. A negative U wave is seen in 10% to 60% of patients with anterior MI, and in up to 30% of patients with inferior MI. Appearance of a negative U wave may precede other ECG changes of infarction by several hours.

## Q Waves

Necrotic tissue has no polarity; thus, with acute myocardial necrosis, the forces of depolarization are not generated in the damaged areas. The remaining forces of ventricular depolarization are accentuated, displacing the mean QRS vector in each lead system away from the zone of necrosis. Thus, the forces of depolarization will be seen moving away, and a Q wave will be recorded.

The lead system closest to the infarcted tissue will record the most significant Q waves. Verily, the reciprocal leads will show initial positive deflection. Although the necrotic area will no longer be capable of depolarization, contraction, or repolarization, it is still surrounded by an area of ischemic myocardium, incompletely depolarized with each ventricular activation.

Note: Significant, pathological Q waves are greater than 0.04 second in duration and at least one fourth of the amplitude of the entire QRS.

In anterior infarction, the foremost change of the QRS complex is the development of a Q wave in the leads that explore the anterior surface (see Figure 12-4).

### Bundle Branch Blocks (BBB) and MI

New BBB (Left or Right) or RBBB and Left anterior hemiblock may accompany acute MI. Overall, about 13% of patients develop a new BBB, and prevalence of LBBB is about the same

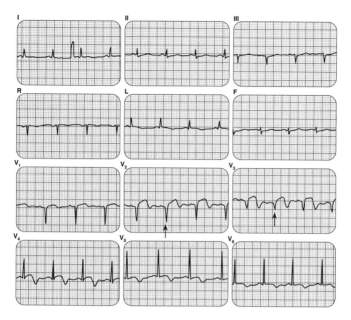

**Figure 12-4**   AWMI.

as RBBB. Blocks that occur with inferior MIs typically resolve, however, blocks that occur with anterior MIs may require a permanent pacemaker. It is important to know that the development of a new BBB with an MI is associated with increased risk for in-hospital death. New LBBB had 34% increased risk, new RBBB had 64% increased risk for death in-hospital. Recall that the diagnosis of MI in patients with LBBB is almost impossible, it is helpful to know if it was preexisting.

### Clinical Significance of Q Waves

In the patient who presents with chest pain and with an ECG showing prior evidence of infarction has a 2.5 times increased mortality rate. Important is past medical history, including risk factors, previous ECG, and family history. Careful review of 12 lead for ST-T changes and QRS configuration is warranted.

### ECG Characteristics

- ST elevation and Q waves are reliable indicators of the anatomic location of injury and infarction in the heart.
- The depth of ST depression, the number of leads demonstrating ST depression, and/or T wave inversion reflect the amount of ischemic heart muscle.
- Q waves may not appear on the ECG until late in the course of infarction, indicating that necrosis has occurred.
- Early in the course of MI, the most prominent ECG finding is ST segment elevation in the lead reflecting the injured tissue.
- A confirming feature is ST depression (reciprocal changes) in the lead opposite the injury.

## Inferior Wall (Diaphragmatic) MI

Inferior wall myocardial infarction (IWMI) usually results from occlusion of the right coronary artery (RCA) (see Figure 12-5).

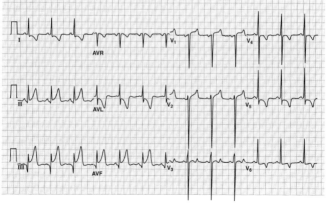

**Figure 12-5**   IWMI.

*ECG Characteristics*
- In the acute phase, ST segment elevation and/or Q waves will be seen in leads II, III and, aVF.
- Also in the acute phase, reciprocal ST segment depression will be seen in leads I, aVL, $V_5$, and $V_6$.
- With further evolution, the ST depression resolves, the T wave is less inverted, but the Q waves persist.
- Eventually, the T waves return to normal, and the fibrotic scar on the inferior wall is represented by Q waves.

Two aspects of IWMI deserve emphasis at this point:

1. With Q waves in leads II, III, and aVF, the mean axis of depolarization may be shifted to the left, more negative than −30°. In the setting of IWMI with leftward shift of axis, left anterior hemiblock cannot be diagnosed.
2. A Q wave in standard lead III may be entirely normal and thus always must be interpreted in light of electro-cardiographic changes seen in standard leads II and aVF. The Q wave in these two leads must be 0.04 second in duration and 25% of the amplitude of the R wave to be considered diagnostic for myocardial damage.

ST elevation in the inferior leads only occurs when proximal right coronary disease exists. Elevated T waves in the inferior leads are seen in distal right coronary disease. Inverted T waves appear in inferior leads with distal left circumflex disease.

### Clinical Significance

All abnormal inferior wall ECG tracings require the analysis of the right precordial leads. Of critical importance is the analysis of $V_{4R}$ to identify the following:

1. The affected coronary artery
2. Presence of right ventricular wall infarction
3. Presence of an AV nodal conduction defect

Other clinical implications include observation for

1. Inappropriate sinus bradycardia
2. AV conduction defects
3. Hypotension and hypoperfusion
4. Extension to the anterior and/or posterior surface evidenced by leads $V_2$, $V_3$, and $V_4$

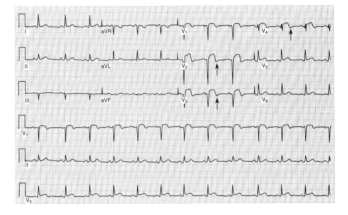

**Figure 12-6**   Antero-septal wall MI.

## Anterior Wall and Antero-Septal Wall MI

Antero-septal wall MI is sometimes called *midanterior MI* (see Figure 12-6).

### ECG Characteristics

- A QS or QR complex in $V_1$ to $V_4$ is diagnostic of an acute anterior wall MI.
- A decrease in the R wave height (excursion) over the anterior precordial leads is also consistent with acute anterior necrosis.

*continues*

*continued*

- Reversed R wave progression, the R wave diminishing from $V_1$ to $V_4$, is often overlooked as a criterion for anterior wall damage.
- With non-Q wave AWMI, look for ST depression with T wave inversion in leads I, aVL, and $V_6$ but no significant alteration of the QRS configuration.

### Clinical Significance

The magnitude of antero-septal or anterior MI may be judged by the extent of the precordial leads involved. Anterior infarctions frequently involve a large area of myocardium; therefore, complications include the following:

1. Cardiogenic shock
2. Sympathetic hyperactivity resulting in sinus tachycardia and hypertension
3. Type II second-degree AV block
4. Complete AV block
5. Left anterior fascicular block
6. Signs of extension to the left lateral wall.

## Anterolateral Wall MI

Anterolateral wall MI is an extensive anterior infarction producing indicative changes across the precordial leads, often involving the ventricular septum (see Figure 12-7).

### ECG Characteristics

- ST elevation, Q waves in I and aVL, but absent in $V_5$ or $V_6$.
- In such instances, all precordial leads should be moved up one intercostal space (high lateral leads). Such a simple manipulation may unmask acute

*continues*

*continued*

infarction changes in $V_5$ and $V_6$ that would otherwise be missed. These criteria are important, because small, insignificant Q waves may be generated in the normal lateral precordial leads, representing septal depolarization in a left-to-right direction.

- Significant Q waves in the lateral precordial leads, $V_2$ to $V_5$, at least 25% of the total amplitude of the QRS complex.

## Clinical Significance

- Loss of wall motion
- Conduction defects in one or more of the fasicles or bundle branches
- Congestive heart failure

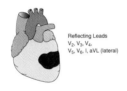

Reflecting Leads
$V_2$, $V_3$, $V_4$,
$V_5$, $V_6$, I, aVL (lateral)

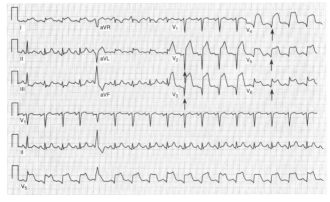

**Figure 12-7**   Anterolateral wall MI.

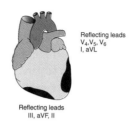

Reflecting leads
$V_4, V_5, V_6$
I, aVL

Reflecting leads
III, aVF, II

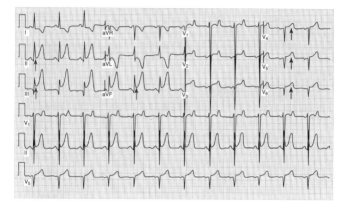

**Figure 12-8** Lateral and inferior wall MI.

## Lateral Wall MI

Lateral wall MI most often results from occlusion of the circumflex artery or results from extensions of AWMI or IWMI (see Figure 12-8).

---

### ECG Characteristics

- ST segment elevation and Q waves in leads I, aVL, $V_5$, and $V_6$
- A drop in QRS amplitude in leads I, aVL, $V_5$, and $V_6$
- Reciprocal ST segment depression may be seen in $V_1$

### Clinical Significance

Once lateral wall MI has been diagnosed, the clinician should be vigilant for changes that may indicate cardiogenic shock or congestive heart failure.

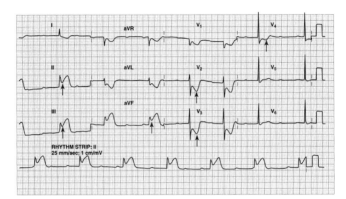

**Figure 12-9**   Posterior wall MI; inferior involvement.

## Posterior Wall MI

Posterior wall MI is caused by occlusion of the dominant RCA or the circumflex artery (see Figure 12-9).

*ECG Characteristics*
- Tall R waves and ST segment depression in leads $V_1$ or $V_2$.
- R wave height greater than S wave depth in lead $V_1$.
- Tall R waves in leads $V_2$, $V_3$ and $V_4$.
- Where there is ST depression in $V_1$ and $V_2$, a true posterior lead would display ST elevation. The posterior ventricular leads, $V_7$–$V_9$, are true views of the posterior surface and should be recorded in clinically suspect patients without 12-lead ECG changes.

*continues*

*continued*

Note: Since criteria for reperfusion therapy require ST elevation in two contiguous leads, the value of a posterior ECG can be significant. If acute changes are documented in the posterior leads, there is justification for reperfusion intervention. Positioning the patient for these leads may be uncomfortable for the patient, and resulting artifact and patient movement may complicate the tracing.

### Clinical Significance

Because the RCA supplies the sinus and AV nodes in most hearts, posterior infarctions are frequently associated with the following:

1. AV conduction defects
2. Changes in sinus rate and rhythm.
3. Signs and symptoms of papillary muscle dysfunction
   a. Cardiogenic shock
   b. Heart failure

## Right Ventricular MI

Right ventricular myocardial infarction is caused by proximal occlusion of the right coronary artery. Although a true right ventricular wall MI can occur independently, it is more commonly associated with IWMI and should be considered in all patients with prolonged CP and no ECG changes. Because the right ventricle is not well represented on a standard ECG, it is critical to perform and interpret right-sided precordial leads in all suspected IWMIs and those MIs complicated with hypotension.

$V_{4R}$ can be easily recorded in the clinical setting. In addition to the correct placement of leads I, II and II, place the V recording electrode on the right side of the chest at the 5th intercostal space, midclavicular line.

*ECG Characteristics*

- ST elevation in right-sided chest leads
- 1 mm or greater ST elevation in lead $V_{4R}$
- A most sensitive indicator of RV infarctions is 0.5 to 1 mm ST elevation in $V_{4R}$

## *Clinical Significance*

Complications of right ventricular MI include

1. Hypotension
2. Decreased cardiac output
3. Cardiogenic shock
4. Jugular venous neck distention
5. Ventricular gallop: $S_3$
6. Summation gallop: $S_3 + S_4$
7. Diminished urine output

Note: These signs may be present without evidence of overt pulmonary congestion.

## Non-Q Wave MI

Absence of Q waves does not rule out MI. Subendocardial infarction may occur without Q waves on the ECG. This is also called non-Q wave MI.

*ECG Characteristics*

- Sub-endocardial injury alters the ST-T wave. Specifically, ST segment depression may drag down the T wave, or the T wave may become inverted as a result of delayed repolarization in the ischemic myocardium.
- In some cases, only small Q waves may appear (less than 5 mm in depth).

*continues*

*continued*

- Diminished R wave amplitude (<10 mm) may appear.
- ST segment elevation, depression, or both may be present, with isolated T wave inversion.
- A representative ECG finding of anterior non-Q wave infarction is a downsloping ST depression, not the typical horizontal ST segment depression seen with posterior MI.
- There will also be an accompanying T wave inversion.

Note: No early ECG changes can predict the evolution of a non-Q wave MI.

### Clinical Significance

1. A high frequency of postinfarction angina is seen.
2. A high frequency of recurrent ischemic events is seen.
3. Patients who present only with T wave changes have a lower mortality than those who present with ST segment depression and T wave changes.

### Summary of ECG Changes Suspicious for Non-Q wave Infarction

1. Inferior wall; leads II, III, and aVF
2. Symmetrical convex ST segment depression on the anterior wall, $V_1$ to $V_4$
3. ST elevation in $V_1$ with ST depression in $V_2$ to $V_4$ without associated posterior wall MI
4. Inverted or biphasic T waves with a terminal inverted segment in $V_2$ and $V_3$
5. Lateral wall; I, aVL, $V_5$, and $V_6$, symmetrical convex ST segment depression
6. Inverted or biphasic T waves

## Non-Classic ECG Presentation of AMI

In the elderly who suffer AMI, the classic ECG changes of ST elevation and reciprocal depression may not be evident early in the process. New-onset atrial fibrillation, with or without chest pain, may herald the infarction. If the clinician has any suspicion after the acute rhythm disturbance, myocardial nuclear imaging, classic changes such as ST elevation on 12-lead ECG and associated elevated enzyme studies may confirm the diagnosis.

ECG complications such as left bundle branch block (LBBB) may mask the ability to confirm MI by 12-lead ECG. In LBBB the initial forces of left-to-right septal activation are no longer intact. So, when AWMI occurs, the resulting Q wave and ST elevation will not be seen in the precordial leads. The left current of flow will overshadow the Q waves seen with IWMI and AWMI. Correlation between clinical presentation and present and previous 12-lead tracings is vital in making this diagnosis.

Table 12-2 provides a quick reference to the surfaces of the heart as seen in leads reflecting those surfaces.

## Proposed Interventions for Suspected MI

Interventions are similar in all instances, the goals being support of airway, oxygenation, heart rate and rhythm, and patient perfusion until reperfusion techniques can be instituted.

MI therapies are evolving as a result of ongoing clinical studies enrolling tens of thousands of patients worldwide. The following interventions are considered for patients with the diagnosis of evolving MI. No implication is made by the order of the listing.

1. Coronary Angioplasty
   a. Percutaneous coronary angioplasty (PCTA) and balloon angioplasty cause barotrauma thus inducing the plaque to be destructed. A major problem is 30% to 35% restenosis of PTCA sites within 6 months of procedure. Aspirin and heparin are given during the

**Table 12-2** The Relationship of Coronary Artery Perfusion to the Sites MI. The Most Effective Lead Systems for Observation and Anticipated Complications

| Coronary artery | Primary area of distribution | Site of infarction and lead system visualization | Anticipated complications |
|---|---|---|---|
| Right | 1. 55% of the SA node<br>2. 90% of the AV node<br>3. Penetrating portion of the bundle of His<br>4. Right atrium and ventricle<br>5. Left inferior surface<br>6. Posterior IV septum<br>7. Left inferior-posterior fascicle | Inferior wall infarction Leads II, III, and aVF | 1. Sinus bradycardia, blocks, and arrest<br>2. AV junctional rhythm<br>3. First-degree AV block<br>4. Second-degree AV block, Type I, Wenckebach<br>5. Complete AV block<br>6. Papillary dysfunction<br>7. Right ventricular wall infarction |
| Left anterior descending | 1. Left anterior wall<br>2. Anterior two thirds of the IV septum<br>3. Bundle of His<br>4. RBBB<br>5. Left anterior-superior fascicle | Left anterior infarction; pre-cordial leads to demon-strate the MI<br>$V_1$ for RBBB<br>Limb leads to observe for conduction defects | 1. Bundle branch blocks<br>2. Type II AV block<br>3. Complete AV block<br>4. Septal defect |
| Left Circumflex | 1. 45% of the SA node<br>2. 10% of the AV node<br>3. Left inferior surface<br>4. Left lateral wall<br>5. Left inferior-posterior fascicle | Left lateral wall infarction Leads I, aVL, and V6 | 1. As in IWMI<br>2. Rupture of the left ventricular free wall<br>3. Ventricular aneurysm<br>4. Papillary dysfunction |

procedure to reduce incidence of acute platelet deposition and thrombosis. However, this endothelial denudation may precipitate acute thrombus formation. Complications are stretching ± tearing and possibly dissection of arterial wall and even aneurysmal dilatation of artery.

b. *Stenting*, the placement of a coil in coronary artery at the position of PTCA. Present studies indicate this may likely be more effective than PTCA for lesions of left anterior descending (LAD) artery. Anti-platelet therapy is recommended to prevent re-occlusion.

c. *Directional Atherectomy*, a routing, auger-type technique, may have improved success in longer lesions. However, it carries an increased risk of dissection, mortality, and MI.

2. Thrombolytic therapy has an overall mortality reduction of 25%. This is of greatest benefit when given within 2 hours (benefit 44%). It is most effective in anterior and Q wave MI. To date, there is no clear benefit for use in unstable angina or non-Q wave MI. Thrombolysis may be achieved if administered in a timely fashion and may be given alone or in combination with heparin and aspirin. Thrombolytic agents include the following:

a. Streptokinase (SK; Kabikinase®, Streptase®)

b. Tissue Plasminogen Activator (TPA, Alteplase®)

c. Reteplase (Retavase®) – recombinant derivative of TPA

d. Anistreplase (APSAC; Eminase®) altepase, streptokinase, reteplase.

3. Platelet Inhibitors – Glycoproteins, predominately platelet inhibitors such as Abciximab (ReoPro®) c7E3 Fab monoclonal antibody against platelet glycoprotein IIb/IIIa, are starting to be used in conjunction with heparin and aspirin. In the Evaluation for Prevention of Ischemic Complications (EPIC) study there was noted an approximate 30% reduction in 30 day death, MI, or need for an emergency procedure for ischemia.

4. Antibiotics – In some patients at risk treatment with Roxithromycin (for Chlamydia pneumoniae organism) after non-Q wave coronary syndromes has resulted in a >50% reduction in recurrent events. Along these theories of infectious causes to thrombus, anti-cytomegalovirus agents also are being evaluated in therapy for atherosclerotic disease.

5. Anti-inflammatory agents also are being assessed for reducing recurrent myocardial ischemic events.

Basic approaches include:

1. ABCs, $O_2$, (P), and IV.
2. Physical assessment and history: Assess HPI, CC, ?chest pain, ?med Hx, ?meds, vital signs, and allergies.
3. Treat the pain with nitroglycerin and/or morphine sulfate according to current therapies.
4. Assess for indicators to perform rapid myocardial perfusion scanning.
5. Evaluate for reperfusion techniques such as thrombolysis.
6. Reassess pain, patient, effect on rate, rhythm, and ectopics if present.
7. Assess cardiac enzymes frequently.
8. Evaluate for conduction defects.
9. Assess hemodynamic status frequently.
10. Assess for s/s congestive heart failure and cardiogenic shock.
11. Assess for AV and bundle branch conduction defects.

## SUMMARY

By current estimates, approximately 1,100,000 people in the United States have a new or recurrent AMI each year. One third prove fatal. Among patients with nonfatal MI, many experience debilitating loss of cardiac muscle because of delay in recognition, diagnosis, and reperfusion.

Despite two decades of pharmacological and percutaneous reperfusion, supported by advances in resuscitation technology, the principal cause of MI morbidity and mortality is still delay from onset of signs and symptoms to recognition and treatment.

Enhancement of prehospital recognition and 12-lead transmission is becoming the standard, the goal being to recognize MI in a timely fashion and intervene to prevent cardiac death. Braunwald suggested that paramedics, nurses, and physicians be educated to recognize candidates for thrombolytic therapy. The concept has been supported since 1990. An algorithm has been developed supporting the use of thrombolytic agents by paramedics in the field and under the direction of a hospital-based physician. Other studies support that premise.

The 12-lead ECG is an invaluable tool but only if in the hands of an educated and observant medical professional. As with any other diagnostic tool, the 12-lead ECG is a beneficial adjunct to thorough history-taking, physical examination, and monitoring of the clinical course.

## REFERENCES

Dobesh, P.P,. & Latham, K.A. (1998). Advancing the battle against acute ischemic syndromes: a focus on the GP IIb-IIIa inhibitors. *Pharmacotherapy, 18,* 663–685.

Epstein, S.E., Speir, E. Zhou, Y.F., et al. (1996). The role of infection in restenosis and atherosclerosis: focus on cytomegalovirus. *Lancet, 348,* (1), s13–s17.

Gurfinkel, E., Bozovich, G., Daroca, A., et al. (1997). Randomized trial of roxithromycin in non Q wave coronary syndrome. *Lancet, 350,* 404.

Holper, E.M., Giugliani, R.P., & Antman, E.M. (1999). Glycoprotein IIb/IIIa inhibitors in acute ST segment elevation myocardial infarction. *Coronary Artery, 10,* 567–573.

Lee, T.H., Rouan, G.W., Weisberg, M.C., et al. (1987). Sensitivity of routine clinical criteria for diagnosing myocardial infarction within 24 hours of hospitalization. *Ann Intern Med., 106,* 181–186.

Moreno, A.M., Alberola, A.G., Tomas, J.G., Chavarri, M.V., Soria, F.C. Sanchez, E.M., & Sanchez, T.G. (1997). Incidence and prognostic significance of right bundle branch block in patients with acute myocardial infarction receiving thrombolytic therapy. *International Journal of Cardiology, 19*, 135–141.

Panju, A.A., Hemmelgarn, B.R., Guyatt, G.H., & Simel, D.L. (1998). Is this patient having a myocardial infarction? *The Journal of the American Medical Association, 280*, 1256–1263.

Plow, E.F., & Byzova, T. (1999). The biology of glycoprotein IIb-IIIa. Joseph J. Jacobs Center for Thrombosis and Vascular Biology, *Coronary Artery Disease, 10*, 547–551.

Ornato, J.P. (1990). The earliest thrombolytic treatment of acute myocardial infarction: ambulance or emergency department? *Clinical Cardiology, 13*, VIII27–31.

# Chapter 13
# Intraventricular Conduction Defects
••••••••••••••••••••••••••••••••••••••••••••••••••••••

An *intraventricular conduction defect* is the result of impaired conduction of electrical impulses through one or more of the divisions of the intraventricular conduction system. The primary conduction pathways that make up the intraventricular conduction system are the right bundle branch and the left main bundle branch (see Figure 13-1). The left main bundle, also known as the common left bundle, divides into fascicles. The primary fascicles are the left anterior fascicle (LAF) and left posterior (LPF) fascicle. Septal fibers, which also extend from the left main branch, vary in length and breadth and are not recognized as true fascicle.s With normal intraventricular depolarization, the right and left ventricles are activated nearly simultaneously (see Figure 13-2).

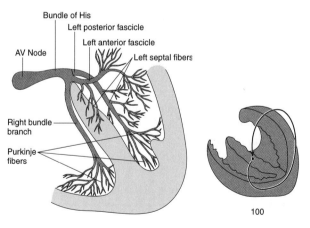

**Figure 13-1**                    **Figure 13-2**

A block at the level of the bundle branches will activate the ventricles in sequence, with the affected bundle depolarizing later. In many instances, depolarization can be delayed so that the QRS duration is greater than 0.10 second.

In bundle branch block, the ventricular activation time (VAT) is altered. VAT is the time from the beginning of the initial inscription of the QRS to the point where the impulse arrives under a particular electrode. The deflection produced is called *intrinsicoid* deflection.

1. $V_1$ measures VAT for the right ventricle = 0.02 second
2. $V_6$ measures VAT for the left ventricle = 0.04 second

## TYPES OF INTRAVENTRICULAR CONDUCTION DEFECTS

An intraventricular conduction defect can occur in any one fascicle or combination of fascicles and causes the ventricles to be activated in sequence rather than nearly simultaneously. When conduction through one or more of the bundle branches is impaired, the conduction pattern is delayed. One ventricle can depolarize out of normal sequence, the ramifications of which include abnormal ventricular wall motion.  There are several defects to consider:

1. Right bundle branch block
2. Incomplete right bundle branch block
3. Rate-related right bundle branch block
4. Right bundle branch block and AMI
5. Left bundle branch block
6. Left anterior fascicular block, a.k.a. left anterior hemiblock
7. Left posterior fascicular block, a.k.a. left posterior hemiblock
8. Incomplete left bundle branch block
9. Rate-related left bundle branch block
10. Left bundle branch block with AMI
11. Left anterior fascicular and right bundle branch block
12. Left anterior fascicular block and AMI

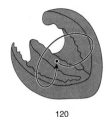

120

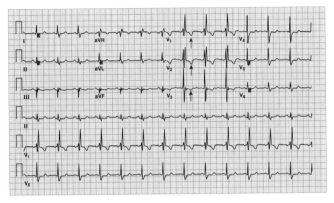

**Figure 13-3** Right bundle branch block.

## Right Bundle Branch Block (RBBB)

Significant alterations in the sequence of right ventricular depolarization occur when the impulse propagation through the right bundle is interrupted. The initial spread of activation is normal during the first 40 ms. In RBBB, the beginning of the QRS complex is usually unchanged so that a small R wave is present in $V_1$ as the wave front crosses the septum; the reciprocal will be a small Q wave in $V_6$. However, when the wave of electrical activity reaches the right bundle (under $V_1$), the normal rapid conduction is halted. To depolarize the right ventricle, the impulse must travel through myocardial tissue rather than specialized conduction pathways, which takes more time. The QRS, then, will represent terminal conduction delay in the form of a broad S wave in leads I, II, $V_5$, and $V_6$ (see Figure 13-3).

### Possible Causes

- Normal variant when rate-related
- Acute heart failure especially RV failure
- Anterior MI
- Cardiomyopathy
- Chagas's disease
- Congenital lesions
- Hypertension
- Ischemic disease
- Lenègre's disease, degenerating conduction pathways
- Lev's disease, calcification/fibrosis of conducting pathways
- Lung disease to include COPB, pulmonary hypotension
- Rheumatic heart disease
- Sleep apnea
- Surgical correction of tetralogy of Fallot
- Surgical correction of a ventricular septal defect
- Syphilis
- Trauma
- Tumors

### ECG Characteristics

- QRS complex 0.12 second or more
- Triphasic complex, rSR′ in $V_1$ and qRS in $V_6$
- Small q and broad S waves in leads I, aVL, and $V_6$
- ST-T wave changes
- Right axis deviation is rare

### Variations in RBBB

1. Incomplete RBBB—QRS duration of ±0.10 second.
2. Rate-related RBBB—RBBB pattern when the sinus rate increases. This is transient, since the QRS will appear normal at 0.10 second once the rate slows.

### Clinical Significance

1. May be a normal variant.
2. In the setting of acute anteroseptal MI, observe for left anterior fascicular block and s/s of heart failure.
3. Incomplete RBBB in conditioned athletes is related to an increase in the muscle mass at the tip of the right ventricle. Once the activity is discontinued, the ECG signs of RBBB disappear. Of the reported 14% of athletes affected with this phenomenon, 10% are between 20 and 35 years old.

### Proposed Interventions

1. Be supportive.
2. If the patient is symptomatic with pain, assess ABCs, $O_2$, (P), IV, ?meds, ?med Hx, ?allergies, and assess vital signs.
3. Treat pain according to current standards of care; reassess after each intervention.
4. If associated with a bradycardia, in the setting of AMI, consider transcutaneous or transvenous pacemaker as soon as possible.
5. New onset RBBB in AMI patients receiving thrombolytic therapy is often transient. RBBB has a negative and independent prognostic impact on survival post MI.

### RBBB and AMI

1. RBBB ECG patterns do not conflict with the patterns of infarction. The initial forces of left to right septal activation are intact, so when an MI occurs, the resulting Q waves and ST elevation will be seen.
2. RBBB that occurs within days of anterior wall MI has a high risk of progressing to involve left anterior fascicular block and complete AV block.

Note: If $MCL_1$ or $V_1$ are the monitoring leads, the progressive involvement of the left bundle will be missed, because fascicular block is only diagnosed in the limb leads.

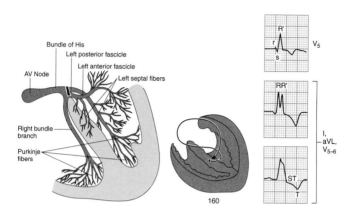

**Figure 13-4** Complete left bundle branch block.

## Left Bundle Branch Block (LBBB)

Complete left bundle branch block (CLBBB) results when there is total interruption of transmission of the electrical impulse through the left main bundle or of the two main branches of the left bundle (see Figure 13-4).

### Possible Causes

- Occlusion in the left main branch or a simultaneous block in both anterior and posterior fascicles
- Usually the result of left anterior descending coronary artery disease
- Acute heart failure
- AMI
- Cardiomyopathy
- Congenital lesions
- Ischemic left coronary artery (LCA) disease
- Lenègre's Disease
- Lev's disease
- Rheumatic heart disease
- Syphilis

- Trauma
- Tumors

---

### ECG Characteristics of CLBBB

In CLBBB, transmission of the impulse to the left ventricle occurs through excitation of the right septal mass; thus, the activation wave crosses the intraventricular septum in a right-to-left direction. Left axis deviation is usually seen in the presence of conduction disease.

---

### ECG Characteristics of LBBB

- QRS greater than 0.12 second
- QS or rS complexes in $V_1$
- R wave in AVR
- Monophasic wide R wave in I, aVL, $V_1$, $V_5$, and $V_6$
- No Q or S waves in leads I, aVL, or $V_6$
- QRS notched or slurred
- VAT exceeds 0.02 second in $V_1$ and 0.04 second in $V_6$
- Secondary ST-T wave abnormalities frequently seen in the left precordial leads, $V_5$, and $V_6$

---

### Variations of CLBBB

1. Incomplete LBBB—QRS duration off ±0.10 second and VAT less than 0.04 second in $V_6$ (controversial).
2. Rate-related LBBB—LBBB pattern when the sinus rate increases. This is transient, since the QRS will appear normal at 0.10 second once the rate slows.

### Clinical Significance

1. May be a normal variant.
2. In the setting of acute anteroseptal MI, observe for s/s of heart failure.

3. Pacemaker induced QRS may have a BBB pattern because the pacer generates an impulse from the right ventricle.

### Proposed Interventions

1. Be supportive.
2. If the patient is symptomatic with pain, assess ABCs, $O_2$, (P), IV, vital signs, ?meds, ?med Hx, and ?allergies.
3. Treat pain according to current standards of care.
4. Assess for AMI and consider therapeutic interventions.
5. Reassess after each intervention.
6. If associated with a bradycardia, in the setting of AMI, consider pacemaker.

### LBBB and AMI

1. LBBB ECG patterns conflict with the patterns of infarction. In LBBB, the initial forces of left bundle branches are incapable of conduction, so depolarization of the right ventricle will appear first, followed by the left. Therefore, if any Q waves originate because of left ventricular MI, the resulting Q waves and ST elevation will not be seen.
2. Upright T wave in $V_5$ and $V_6$ may indicate ischemia in that area.
   a. This is because in LBBB, the ST segment and T wave are usually opposite in polarity from the terminal portion of the QRS.
   b. When the ST segment and T wave are of the same polarity as the terminal portion of the QRS, this is an acute sign of possible ischemia.
3. R wave amplitude may decrease over left ventricular leads.
4. Q waves in I, aVL, or $V_6$ greater than 0.04 second may indicate anteroseptal or lateral wall MI.
5. There may be ST segment and T wave displacement and loss of normal ST segment convex appearance.

Although these changes may be useful indicators, there is no conclusive way to diagnose an AMI in the presence of LBBB. The presence of LBBB should itself alert the clinician to the possibility of an MI, because this commonly accompanies an anterior wall MI.

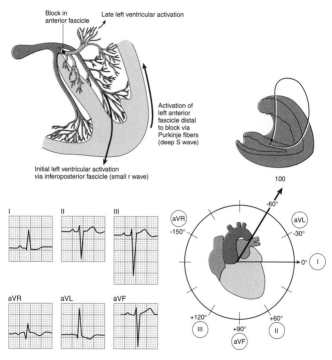

**Figure 13-5**   Left anterior fascicular block.

### Fascicular Blocks

The main left bundle divides early into the anterior-superior and the posterior-inferior branches. The blood supply to the left anterior fascicle is from the septal branch of the left anterior descending coronary artery. The posterior fascicle has two blood supplies and is not as vulnerable as the anterior division (see Figure 13-5).

### Possible Causes

- Normal variant in asthemic body types
- Congenital
- Anterior MI (most common)
- Aortic valve disease
- Arterial occlusion
- Cardiomyopathy
- Hypertensive heart disease
- Hyperkalemia
- Ischemic heart disease
- Lenègre's disease
- Lev's disease
- Occasionally with IWMI
- Following surgical correction for tetralogy of Fallot

### ECG Characteristics

- QRS complex usually at 0.10 second and increased voltage
- Left axis deviation (–40°) or more
- rS in leads II, III, and aVF; no terminal R wave, rS in $V_6$
- Small Q waves in leads I and aVL due to the shift of initial forces inferiorly and to the right
- A terminal r or R that occurs in aVR

### Clinical Significance

1. Monitor for bifascicular (RBBB and left anterior or fascicular block [LAFB])
2. Monitor for complete heart block

### Proposed Interventions

1. Be supportive.
2. If the patient is symptomatic with pain, assess ABCs, $O_2$, (P), IV, vital signs, ?meds, ?med Hx, and ?allergies.

3. Treat pain according to current standards of care.
4. Assess for etiology and initiate appropriate interventions. Be suspicious of AMI.
5. Reassess after each intervention.
6. If associated with a bradycardia, in the setting of AMI, consider a pacemaker.

## LAFB and RBBB

LAFB, also referred to as LAH, can occur with RBBB because they are similar in structure and share much of the same blood supply. The phenomenon is recognized as RBBB in $V_1$, and if the S wave is greater than the R wave, then left axis deviation is present. When RBBB is concomitant with an LAFB, it is called *bifascicular block*. Often, the LAFB obscures the RBBB.

---

### *ECG Characteristics*
- QRS complex usually at 0.10 second
- RBBB pattern with left axis deviation (RBBB + LAFB)
- RBBB pattern with right axis deviation (RBBB + left posterior fascicular block [LPFB])

---

### *Proposed Interventions*
1. Be supportive.
2. If the patient is symptomatic with pain, assess ABCs, $O_2$, (P), IV, vital signs, ?meds, ?med Hx, and ?allergies.
3. Treat pain according to current standards of care.
4. Assess for etiology and initiate appropriate interventions.
5. Reassess after each intervention.
6. If associated with a bradycardia, in the setting of AMI, consider a pacemaker.

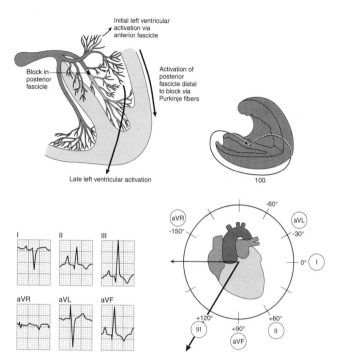

**Figure 13-6**   Left posterior fascicular block.

## Left Posterior Fascicular Block (LPFB)

Isolated LPFB, because the left fascicle is shorter and thicker than the anterior fascicle and has a dual blood supply. However, LPFB is more serious, because it implies compromise to both blood supplies and damage to the inferior conduction system. The impulse activates the ventricle via the left anterior superior fascicle, which produces the characteristic right axis deviation (see Figure 13-6).

### Possible Causes

- AMI
- Aortic valve calcification

- Cardiomyopathy
- Ischemic heart disease
- Lenègre's disease
- Lev's disease

---

### ECG Characteristics
- QRS complex usually at 0.10 second
- Right axis deviation (+120°) or more
- Q wave in leads II, III, and aVF
- r wave in leads I and aVL
- Increased QRS voltage in limb leads

---

### Clinical Significance

1. Rarely a normal variant.
2. In the setting of acute anteroseptal MI, observe for s/s of heart failure.

### Proposed Interventions

1. Be supportive.
2. If the patient is symptomatic with pain, assess ABCs, $O_2$, (P), IV, vital signs, ?meds, ?med Hx, and ?allergies.
3. Treat pain according to current standards of care.
4. Assess for etiology and initiate appropriate interventions.
5. Reassess after each intervention.
6. If associated with a bradycardia, in the setting of AMI, consider a pacemaker.

## Trifascicular Block

When a block is located in each of the three main fascicles on the bundle branch system, it is called *trifascicular block*. If the block is complete, the patient will be left with an escape ventricular pacemaker, below the lesions. Accuracy of ECG diagnosis of trifascicular block is only 50%. Confirmation requires electrophysiologic evaluation.

If the block is incomplete, then the supraventricular impulses will encounter AV delay, revealed as first-degree or second-degree Type II AV block.

Analyzing the ECG involves assessing leads II, III, and aVF for axis shift with LAFB as well as assessing the PR interval and signs of complete AV block. $V_1$ should always be assessed for RBBB.

### Possible Causes

- Coronary artery disease
- Lenègre's disease
- Lev's disease

### ECG Characteristics

- rS in leads II, III, and aVF; No terminal R wave
- Small Q waves in lead I and aVL due to the shift of initial forces inferiorly and to the right
- A terminal r or R that occurs in aVR

In addition, trifascicular block can present with complete AV block with idioventricular rhythm. Also, trifascicular block can appear with any of the following combinations:

1. RBBB with LAFB and first- or second-degree (Type I or II) AV block
2. RBBB with LPFB and first- or second-degree (Type I or II) AV block
3. LBBB with first or second degree (Type I or II) AV block

### Clinical Significance

Trifascicular block is significant, because it results in profound bradycardia with hypotension and hypoperfusion. There is a high rate of progress to complete AV block in patients with trifascicular block.

### Proposed Interventions

1. Be supportive.
2. If the patient is symptomatic with pain, assess ABCs, $O_2$, (P), IV, vital signs, ?meds, ?med Hx, and ?allergies.
3. Treat pain according to current standards of care.
4. Assess for etiology and initiate appropriate interventions.
5. Reassess after each intervention.
6. Prepare for pacemaker insertion.

Table 13-1 summarizes conduction abnormalities of the left bundle, indicating the site of the conduction defect, the direction of the QRS axis, and the duration of the QRS complex.

**Table 13-1** Summary of Conduction Abnormalities of the Left Bundle, Indicating the Site of the Conduction Defect, the Direction of the QRS Axis, and the Duration of the QRS Complex

| Conduction defect | Site of the defect | Axis | QRS duration |
|---|---|---|---|
| Left anterior fascicular block | Anterior-superior branch | Greater than −45° | 0.12 second or less |
| Left posterior fascicular block | Posterior-inferior branch | Greater than +100° | 0.12 second or less |
| Complete left bundle branch block | Left main | Less than −30° | 0.14 second or more |
| Complete left bundle branch block with left axis deviation | Complete anterior-superior branch | Greater than −45° | 0.14 second or more |
| Complete left bundle branch block with right axis deviation | Complete posterior-inferior branch Partial superior-inferior branch | Greater than +110° | 0.14 second or more |

## SUMMARY

Structure and function are closely related in the human body. The heart is especially revealing when there is the slightest alteration in its electrical system. Without the flow of electric impulses, the muscular pump fails to be effective. The framework of the heart that allows the travel of critical action potentials is structurally revealed by the 12-lead and in many instances the 18-lead ECG to include right ventricular assessment.

Nutrition and oxygenation via arterial blood flow are as important to the intraventricular conduction system as they are to the myocardium. Careful examination for the underlying cause of the conduction defect is as important as treating the effects of the defect. Early recognition of a patient's signs and symptoms should myocardial compromise occur will limit the time to reperfusion and hence increase chances of survival.

# Chapter 14
# Hypertrophy
• • • • • • • • • • • • • • • • • • • • • • • • • • • • • • • • • • • • • • • • • • • • • • • • •

Hypertrophy is an increase in bulk or size of body tissue. Cardiac hypertrophy or chamber enlargement describes the increase in overall size of the atria or ventricles. Hypertrophy is a compensatory mechanism for increased workload such as with chronic heart disease, hypertension, insufficient valves, or stenotic valves. Each chamber is capable of hypertrophy and may affect any or all of the others.

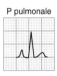

**Figure 14-1** P pulmonale.

### RIGHT ATRIAL ENLARGEMENT

*P pulmonale* describes the increased size, morphology, and duration of P wave that represent RAE (see Figure 14-1).

### Possible Causes

- Atrial septal defect
- Chronic lung disease
- Eisenmenger's syndrome (congenital anomaly with right-to-left shunt)
- Mitral stenosis
- Primary pulmonary disease
- Pulmonary emboli
- Pulmonary stenosis
- Pulmonary vascular hypertension
- Tricuspid insufficiency

**ECG Characteristics**

- P waves: Tall, peaked P waves; (+) in leads I, III, and aVF; sometimes in $V_1$
- P wave morphology: Notched, widened to greater than 0.12 second
- P wave axis: Rightward at about +70° when associated with chronic pulmonary disease
- PR interval: As with the underlying rhythm
- QRS complex: ± 0.10 second; qR in $V_1$ (in the absence of MI); diminished voltage in $V_1$ and increased voltage in $V_2$
  - Rate: As with the underlying rhythm
  - Rhythm: As with the underlying rhythm

## Clinical Significance

RAE is secondary to ventricular hypertrophy, which in turn is a manifestation of a chronic condition.

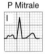
P Mitrale

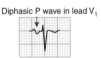
Diphasic P wave in lead $V_1$

**Figure 14-2** P mitrale.

## LEFT ATRIAL ENLARGEMENT (LAE)

*P mitrale* describes the increased size, morphology, and duration of P wave that represent LAE (see Figure 14-2).

## Possible Causes

- Aortic stenosis
- Aortic insufficiency
- Athletics
- Coarctation of the aorta
- Hypertension

- Hypertrophic cardiomyopathy
- MI

---

### ECG Characteristics

- P waves: Tall, peaked P waves; (+) in leads I and II, may be negative in III and aVF
- P wave morphology: Notched, widened to greater than 0.12 second
- P wave axis: Within normal limits
- PR interval: As with the underlying rhythm
- QRS complex: 0.10 second or less
  - Rate: As with the underlying rhythm
  - Rhythm: As with the underlying rhythm

---

### RIGHT VENTRICULAR HYPERTROPHY (RVH)

Left ventricular activity usually overshadows the right, so when RVH is visible on the ECG, the condition is severe (see Figure 14-3). As RVH develops, dilation occurs as well as intrinsic lung disease which leads to increased pulmonary vascular resistance. This may bring about pneumothorax and pulmonary embolism which causes massive pulmonary vasoconstriction. This leads to acute cor pulmonale, right heart failure, hypotension and death.

### Possible Causes

- Pulmonary stenosis
- Tetralogy of Fallot
- Eisenmenger's syndrome
- Mitral insufficiency with pulmonary hypertension
- Mitral stenosis
- Primary pulmonary disease
- Pulmonary vascular hypertension
- Pulmonary emboli
- Pulmonary stenosis
- Sleep apnea

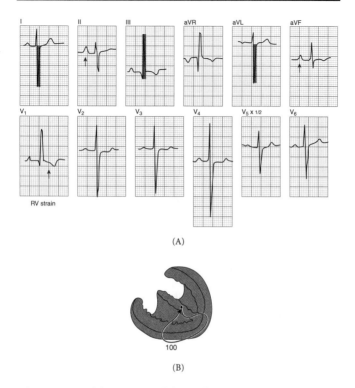

(A)

(B)

**Figure 14-3** (A) RVH 14-3, (B) QRS loop in RVH.

- Tricuspid regurgitation
- Differential of R wave in $V_1$
  a. Normal variant
  b. Right axis deviation (left posterior fascicular block more common than RVH and RBBB)
  c. Pulmonary embolism or hypertension
  d. Wolff Parkinson White syndrome: usually a tall R wave in $V_2$
  e. Posterior extension of the infarction
  f. Duchenne muscular dystrophy

### ECG Characteristics

The most useful clue to RVH is right axis deviation and abnormalities in $V_1$. Recall that $V_1$ faces the right ventricle.

- Early R wave progression (more common than RAD)
- Right axis deviation (RAD)
- R wave height to S wave depth ratio greater than 1 in $V_1$
- R wave equals 7 mm in $V_1$
- S wave equals 7 mm in $V_5$ and $V_6$
- R wave in $V_1$ plus the S wave in $V_5$ or $V_6$ is greater than 10 mm
- rSr with R wave greater than 10 mm, or qRS pattern in $V_1$
- Right ventricular strain pattern
- Secondary ST-T changes; T wave inversion in AVF
- Associated right atrial enlargement

### LEFT VENTRICULAR HYPERTROPHY (LVH)

The QRS complex depicted on a normal ECG represents depolarization of the ventricles and reflects left ventricular muscle mass. It follows, then, that left ventricular enlargement will be represented on the ECG by changes in the duration of the QRS complex in some of the leads and axis deviation (see Figure 14-4). Secondary ST-T changes and left atrial changes in P wave are present.

### Possible Causes

- Systolic overload
  a. Aortic stenosis/insufficiency
  b. Coarctation of the aorta
  c. Systemic hypertension
  d. Hypertrophic cardiomyopathy

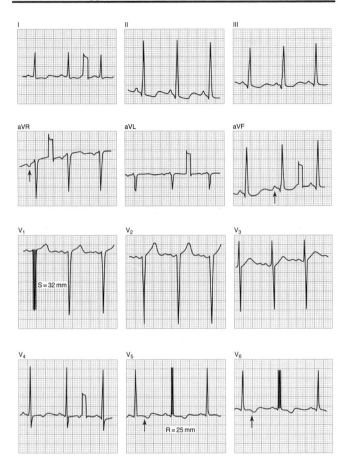

**Figure 14-4** LVH $SV_1$+ $RV_6$ = greater than 45 mm.

- Diastolic overload
  a. Aortic/mitral regurgitation
  b. Ventricular septal defects
- Primary pulmonary disease
- Athletics

### ECG Characteristics

There are several methods to assess the ECG determinants of LVH. These include the following:

- Voltage
  a. Mean QRS vector
  b. Index of Lewis
- Sokolow-Lyon
- Cornell voltage test

ECG findings that warrant further assessment and confirmation for LVH include the following:

- QRS vector: Leftward and more posterior, greater than $-30°$
- QRS duration: 0.10 second or less
- QRS morphology: Unchanged
- Axis: $-30°$; greater when bundle branch block is present with myocardial fibrosis secondary to hypertension.

## Voltage Criteria

There are several ways to determine the presence of LVH by using the 12-lead ECG. Many elaborate point systems have been developed for LVH identification. It is always best to work with a method that uses two levels of certainty, such as (1) voltage criteria plus (2) secondary ST-T changes.

Do not be resigned to using only one criterion. Adapting to the patient's circumstance requires consideration of many variables. Caution: Use of voltage criteria alone can also result in a false negative identification.

1. Mean QRS vector: R wave greater than 27 mm in $V_5$ or greater than 25 mm in $V_6$. (This application has merit for patients older than 35 years.)
2. Index of Lewis (T): Add the net positive deflection in lead I in millimeters plus the net negative deflection in lead III in millimeters. A sum greater than 21 mm indicates LVH.

3. Lewis (T) criteria corrects for left anterior fascicular block (LAFB): The height of the R wave: R wave in aVL should measure greater than 13 mm.

4. Sokolow-Lyon criteria: This method is very popular but is not recommended for patients under the age of 35 years.
   a. Look at leads $V_1$, $V_5$, and $V_6$.
   b. When the S wave in $V_1$ plus the R wave in $V_5$ or $V_6$ is 35 mm or greater, it is positive for LVH. ($SV_1 + RV_5$ or $RV_6$ = greater than 35mm indicates LVH.)

5. Voltage criteria
   a. The R wave in aVL is greater than 11 mm.
   b. The S wave in $V_1$ plus the R wave in $V_5$ or the R wave in $V_6$ is greater than 35 mm. Or,
   c. The R wave in $V_5$ or $V_6$ is greater than 25 mm. The specificity is greater than 95% when using this criteria, but the sensitivity is low, less than 30%.

6. Cornell voltage test: R wave in aVL + S wave in $V_3$ = greater than 28 mm in males and 20 mm in females.

## VENTRICULAR STRAIN PATTERN

*Ventricular strain* denotes ST segment and T wave changes that are frequently seen with ventricular hypertrophy. The reason for these changes is not clear. It is thought that conduction delays through the thickened walls play an important role as does ischemia, due to the increased demand caused by increased muscle fiber diameter (see Figure 14-5).

### ECG Characteristics

Secondary ST-T wave changes are sometimes referred to as left ventricular strain pattern:

- Sagging ST segments and inverted T waves in every lead with a tall R wave
- A rising ST and upright T in every lead with a deep S wave

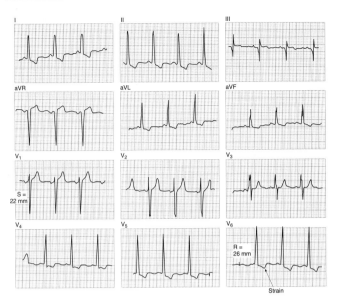

**Figure 14-5** Left ventricular strain pattern.

## Clinical Significance

Hypertension is the leading cause of left ventricular strain. Second is left ventricular volume overload. If the strain is secondary to aortic insufficiency the patient may require aortic valve replacement. Once the etiology of the hypertrophy has been confirmed, treatment is directed to the underlying cause.

## Proposed Interventions

Interventions are directed to supporting the patient's airway, oxygenation, managing heart rate and rhythm, perfusion and controlling hypertension.

## SUMMARY

The 12-lead ECG reveals information about all four of the heart's chambers and allows the clinician to interpret nonacute conditions. The assessment of increased amplitude can support the diagnosis of chamber enlargement due to chronic disease. The 12-lead ECG is a valuable tool in diagnosing the existence of chamber hypertrophy. Awareness of the existence of chamber abnormality may alter the choice of intervention and affect long-term outcome.

# Appendix A
# Medication Profiles

........................................................

> **Premise**
>
> To know a drug, when to use it, what to expect and, most important, when NOT to use it, is a key to the intervention and care of the patient in cardiac compromise.

## INTRODUCTION

The purpose of this appendix is to review common medications used in the care of patients with cardiovascular disease. This is a quick reference only, and is not all-inclusive; knowledge of the pharmacokinetics should be maintained with intense study and review of pharmacological references. Also, practitioners should be aware of current standards, guidelines, and oversight that guide patient care in their specific environment.

## ABCIXIMAB

| | |
|---|---|
| Generic Name: | abciximab |
| Trade Names: | Reopro® |
| Classes: | antiplatelet agent, glycoprotein (GP) IIb/IIIa inhibitor |
| Standard Supply: | 2.0 mg/1.0 ml in 5.0 ml vial (must be refrigerated) |

Mechanism of Action:

* reversibly binds with GP IIb/IIIa receptors on the surface of platelets, by inhibiting the binding of fibrinogen, von Willebrant factor, and other adhesive molecules. Binding with GP IIb/IIIa receptors effec-

tively prevents formation of intravascular thrombus and may contribute to the resolution of preexisting thrombus.

**Indications:**

- adjunctive to, or in preparation for, percutaneous transluminal coronary angioplasty (PTCA) for the prevention and management of acute coronary syndrome and associated acute cardiac ischemic complications in patients at risk for abrupt closure of the treated coronary vessel. Includes intravenous infusion monitoring during prehospital interfacility transportation.
- thrombotic arterial disease

**Contraindications:**

- active internal bleeding or recent history (within 30 days) of clinically significant gastrointestinal or genitourinary bleeding
- history of stroke with current residual neurological deficit, or within the past two years
- bleeding disorder, condition, or predisposition
- concomitant use of Coumadin® (warfarin), or use within the past 7 days unless prothrombin time is <1.2 times control
- thrombocytopenia (<100,000 cells/μl)
- trauma or major surgery within the past 6 weeks
- intracranial neoplasm
- arteriovenous malformation, aneurysm, or evidence of aortic dissection
- severe uncontrolled hypertension (systolic blood pressure >180 mm Hg/diastolic blood pressure >110 mm Hg)
- history of vasculitis
- concomitant use of another GP IIb/IIIa inhibitor
- acute pericarditis

- concomitant use of IV Dextran® (results in a high incidence of bleeding)
- known hypersensitivity to abciximab or murine proteins

**Adverse Reactions:**

- bleeding
- hemorrhagic stroke and intracranial bleeding
- thrombocytopenia

The most common sites of spontaneous bleeding include venous and arterial access sites. Major bleeding has been demonstrated to occur more often in patients who are >65 years old, <75 kg, with a history of gastrointestinal disease, and patients receiving thrombolytics or heparin.

**NOTES ON ADMINISTRATION**

- Heparin should be concomitantly administered and monitored with abciximab.
- Due to the risk of spontaneous bleeding during administration of abciximab, the following procedures should be avoided whenever possible: arterial and venous punctures, intramuscular injection, placement of a urinary catheter, placement of a nasogastric tube, and nasotracheal intubation.

**Routes of Administration:**

- IVPush
- continuous intravenous infusion

**Onset of Action:**

- several minutes

**Drug Interactions:**

- other medications that affect hemostasis: thrombolytics, oral anticoagulants, aspirin and other nonsteroidal anti-inflammatory drugs (NSAIDs), dipyridamole, ticlopidine, and clopidogrel
- herbal products containing ginkgo, biloba, ginger, and garlic

**Adult Dosage:**

- 0.25 mg/kg slow IVPush over 5 minutes then

*if the patient weighs <80 kg:*

- 0.125 µg/kg/minute (0.09 mg/kg) intravenous infusion

*if the patient weighs >80 kg:*

- 10 µg/minute (7.2 mg) in 250 ml of D5W or normal saline 21 ml/hour for 12 hours

**Caveats:**

Weight-based dosing of abciximab and concomitant heparin are essential to decrease the incidence of bleeding. An infusion pump is required for intravenous infusion administration of abciximab. Abciximab infusions must be administered through a low-protein binding 0.2 or 0.22 micron in-line filter.


## ACETYLSALICYLIC ACID (ASA)

| | |
|---|---|
| **Generic Name:** | acetylsalicylic acid (ASA) |
| **Trade Names:** | Aspirin®, Bayer®, Excedrin®, Bufferin®, Goldline Children's Chewable Aspirin®, others |
| **Classes:** | platelet aggregator inhibitor, analgesic, antipyretic, anti-inflammatory |

**Mechanism of Action:**

- blocks formation of thromboxane $A_2$, which prevents platelet clumping and blood clot formation (specifically in the coronary arteries)

**Indications:**

- chest pain consistent with an AMI
- prevention and treatment of unstable angina (USA)

**Contraindications:**

- bleeding disorders
- known hypersensitivity to the medication

**Adverse Reactions:**

- gastrointestinal irritation
- gastrointestinal bleeding

## NOTES ON ADMINISTRATION

**Route of Administration:**

- oral (chewed or swallowed)

**Onset of Action:**

- 20–30 minutes

**Drug Interactions:**

- none in an emergency setting

**Adult Dosage:**

- 325 mg tablet *or*
- up to four 81 mg children's flavored chewable tablets or
- administer this medication according to current standards and guidelines

### ADENOSINE

| | |
|---|---|
| **Generic Name:** | adenosine |
| **Trade Name:** | Adenocard® |
| **Classes:** | antiarrhythmic, endogenous nucleoside |
| **Standard Supply:** | 6.0 mg/2.0 ml |

**Mechanism of Action:**

- slows conduction of electrical impulses through the SA node and node
- interrupts reentry pathways and can terminate paroxysmal SVT (PSVT)

**Indications:**

- PSVT, including that caused by WPW syndrome refractory to common vagal maneuvers
- wide complex tachycardia of uncertain origin after administering lidocaine

**Contraindications:**
- second-degree block
- complete (third-degree) block
- Sick-sinus syndrome
- known hypersensitivity to the drug

**Adverse Reactions:**
- transient flushing of the skin
- chest pain
- dyspnea
- brief period of asystole or bradycardia
- hemodynamic instability

## NOTES ON ADMINISTRATION

**Onset of Action:**
- seconds (adenosine has a 5–10 second half-life)

**Drug Interactions:**
- concomitant use of methylxanthines may inhibit desired effects
- concomitant use of carbamazepine (Tegretol) can create high degree of AV block
- higher doses may be necessary when theophylline has been taken

**Adult Dosage:**
- 6.0 mg rapid IVP followed by rapid infusion of normal saline
- if the rhythm does not convert within 2 minutes, administer 12 mg rapid IVP followed by rapid infusion of normal saline
- if the rhythm does not convert within 2 minutes after the second dose, administer 12 mg rapid IVP followed by a rapid fluid infusion of normal saline

## AMIODARONE HCl

| | |
|---|---|
| **Generic Name:** | amiodarone HCl |
| **Trade Names:** | Cordarone®, Pacerone® |
| **Class:** | antiarrhythmic class III |
| **Standard Supply:** | 150 mg/3.0 ml |

**Mechanism of Action:**

- Antiarrhythmic, potent vasodilator
- prolongs action potential
- prolongs effective refractory period in all cardiac tissue including accessory pathways
- noncompetitive block of alpha- and beta-adrenergic receptors
- reduces heart rate through beta-blocking effects
- blocks sodium, potassium, and calcium channels
- paroxysmal atrial fibrillation with rapid ventricular response

**Indications:**

- recurring ventricular fibrillation
- recurring unstable ventricular tachycardia
- prophylaxis of recurring ventricular fibrillation and unstable ventricular tachycardia

**Contraindications:**

- because toxicities are common, severe, and irreversible, this medication should be considered after other antiarrhythmics have been shown to be ineffective
- known hypersensitivity to the medication
- SA node dysfunction
- marked sinus bradycardia
- second-degree heart block
- complete (third-degree) heart block
- cardiogenic shock
- electrolyte imbalance (hypocalcemia, hypomagnesemia)
- thyroid disease

**Adverse Reactions:**

- hypotension
- pulmonary toxicity and fibrosis
- asystole/cardiac arrest/PEA
- bradycardia
- atrioventricular block
- torsades de pointes
- congestive heart failure

## NOTES ON ADMINISTRATION

**Route of Administration:**

- intravenous infusion
- po

**Onset of Action:**

- various response

**Drug Interactions:**

- none in the emergency setting
- concomitant use of beta-blockers or calcium-channel blockers
- concomitant use of digoxin and procainamide causes an additive effect

**Adult Dosage:**

- 150 mg rapid IV infusion over 10 minutes, then add 3.0 ml of the medication (150 mg) to 100 ml of D5W and rapidly infuse
- 360 mg slow IV infusion over the next 6 hours

### ATROPINE SULFATE

| | |
|---|---|
| **Generic Name:** | atropine sulfate |
| **Trade Name:** | Atropine® |
| **Class:** | anticholinergic |
| **Standard Supply:** | • 1.0 mg/10 ml |
| | • 8.0 mg/20 ml |

**Mechanism of Action:**

- blocks or antagonizes the effects of acetylcholine, thus inhibiting parasympathetic stimulation

**Systemic Effects:**

- decreases salivary and gastrointestinal secretions/motility
- causes bronchodilation
- decreases mucous production
- decreases urinary bladder tone
- causes mydriasis (pupillary dilation)
- decreases sweat production

**Cardiac Effects:**

- increases the rate of SA node discharge
- enhances conduction through the node

**Indications:**

- hemodynamically significant bradycardia
- asystole
- PEA with ventricular rate less than 60 per minute
- narrow-complex second-degree block
- narrow-complex complete (third-degree) block
- antidote for cholinergic poisonings (e.g., organophosphate and carbamates)

**Contraindications:**

- wide complex second-degree (Type II) block
- wide complex complete (third-degree) block

**Adverse Reactions:**

- tachycardia
- anxiety
- palpitations
- headache
- blurred vision

- delirium
- dry mouth
- dilated pupils

## NOTES ON ADMINISTRATION
### Routes of Administration
- IVP
- ET

### Onset of Action:
- 1 minute

### Drug Interaction:
- sodium bicarbonate inactivates

### Adult Dosage:
- for hemodynamically significant bradycardia: 0.5–1.0 mg IVP or 1.0–2.5 mg ET every 3–5 minutes to a total dose of 3.0 mg or 0.03–0.04 mg/kg
- for asystole and slow PEA: 1.0 mg IVP or 2.0–2.5 mg ET every 3–5 minutes to a total dose of 3.0 mg or 0.03–0.04 mg/kg
- for cholinergic poisonings: 2.0–5.0 mg IVP every 5–10 minutes, or administer this medication according to local protocol

NOTE: For adult ET administration, deliver 2.0–2.5 times the recommended IVP dose and dilute with normal saline according to protocol.

## BRETYLIUM TOSYLATE

| | |
|---|---|
| **Generic Name:** | bretylium tosylate |
| **Trade Name:** | Bretylol® |
| **Class:** | antiarrhythmic |
| **Standard Supply:** | • 500 mg/5.0 ml |
| | • 500 mg/10 ml |

**Mechanism of Action:**

- elevates ventricular fibrillation threshold
- suppresses ventricular ectopy
- may convert ventricular fibrillation or ventricular tachycardia to a supraventricular rhythm

NOTE: Bretylium initially causes a slight increase in heart rate, blood pressure, and cardiac output. These sympathomimetic effects last approximately 20 minutes in the noncardiac arrest setting. Then, norepinephrine release is inhibited, which results in an adrenergic blockade. Hypotension may develop, particularly orthostatic hypotension.

**Indications:**

- ventricular fibrillation and pulseless ventricular tachycardia refractory to first-line  antiarrhythmics
- ventricular tachycardia with a pulse refractory to first-line antiarrhythmics
- PVCs refractory to first-line antiarrhythmics

**Contraindication:**

- none in the emergency setting

**Adverse Reactions:**

- hypotension
- nausea and vomiting
- dizziness
- syncope
- seizures
- chest pain
- bradycardia

## NOTES ON ADMINISTRATION
**Routes of Administration:**

- IVP
- intravenous infusion

**Onset of Action:**
- 5 minutes

**Drug Interactions:**
- digoxin (Lanoxin®) causes increased hypotension
- sodium bicarbonate inactivates

**Adult Dosage:**
- for cardiac arrest: 5.0 mg/kg IVP to a maximum dose of 35 mg/kg
- for a conscious patient with arrhythmias: dilute the bolus amount in 50 ml or 100 ml of normal saline and infuse over 10–15 minutes

## CALCIUM CHLORIDE

| | |
|---|---|
| **Generic Name:** | calcium chloride |
| **Trade Name:** | Calcium Chloride® |
| **Class:** | electrolyte |
| **Standard Supply:** | 1.0 g/10 ml |

**Mechanism of Action:**
- increases myocardial contractility
- increases ventricular automaticity

**Indications:**
- calcium-channel blocker toxicity (e.g., verapamil, nifedipine)
- acute hyperkalemia (e.g., renal failure with cardiovascular compromise)
- magnesium sulfate toxicity
- acute hypocalcemia
- black widow spider envenomation

**Contraindication:**
- none in the emergency setting

**Adverse Reactions:**

- arrhythmias
- hypotension
- syncope
- bradycardia
- nausea and vomiting
- cardiac arrest

## NOTES ON ADMINISTRATION

**Route of Administration:**

- IVP

**Onset of Action:**

- immediate

**Drug Interactions:**

- sodium bicarbonate inactivates
- thoroughly flush IV tubing with normal saline before and after administration of this medication

**Adult Dosage:**

- 2.0–4.0 mg/kg IVP
- repeat 2.0–4.0 mg/kg IVP every 10 minutes *or*
- administer this medication according to current standards and guidelines

## DIAZEPAM

| | |
|---|---|
| **Generic Name:** | diazepam |
| **Trade Name:** | Valium® |
| **Classes:** | anticonvulsant, sedative |
| **Standard Supply:** | 10 mg/2.0 ml |

**Mechanism of Action:**

- inhibits neuronal transmission in the central nervous system
- causes muscle relaxation

**Indications:**

- major motor seizures
- status epilepticus
- sedation before cardioversion or external transthoracic pacing
- skeletal muscle relaxation
- acute anxiety state
- alcohol withdrawal syndrome
- diazepam is a benzodyazepam that is used clinically as a hypnotic

**Contraindication:**

- known hypersensitivity to the medication

**Adverse Reactions:**

- hypotension
- respiratory depression or arrest
- blurred vision
- nausea and vomiting
- drowsiness

## NOTES ON ADMINISTRATION

**Routes of Administration:**

- immediate (IVP)
- IM and rectal (varies)

**Onset of Action:**

- IVP
- IM

**Drug Interactions:**

- incompatible with many medications

**Adult Dosage:**

- administer under current standards and guidelines

## DILTIAZEM HCl

| | |
|---|---|
| **Generic Name:** | diltiazem HCl |
| **Trade Names:** | Cardizem® |
| **Classes:** | calcium-channel blocker, slow channel blocker, calcium antagonist (non-dihydropyridine, benzodiazepine calcium-channel blocker) |
| **Standard Supply** | • 5.0 mg/1.0 ml in 5.0 ml and 10 ml vials (requires refrigeration) |

**Mechanism of Action:**

- depresses contractility, impulse conduction, and automaticity in myocardial and vascular smooth muscle (reduced peripheral vascular resistance) (due to inhibiting the movement of calcium ions across the cell membranes of specialized contractile cells, specifically through slow calcium channels)
- decreases sino-atrial and atrioventricular conduction (this prolongs the atrial-His-Purkinje refractory period, which prolongs PR interval and decreases heart rate)
- increased cardiac output in the presence of supraventricular tachyarrhythmias
- calcium channel antagonism may dilate coronary vasculature (results in increased blood flow and oxygen delivery, of particular value in vasospastic conditions)
- reduces blood pressure (due to dilation of peripheral arterioles and negative inotropy or depressed contractility)
- reduces afterload (due to dilation of peripheral arterioles and negative inotropy or depressed contractility)

**Indications:**

- rate reduction and control of atrial fibrillation, atrial flutter, and PSVT
- unstable angina
- severe hypertension

**Contraindications:**
- sick sinus syndrome
- second-degree AV block
- hypotension (systolic blood pressure <100 mm Hg)
- AMI
- concomitant use of a beta blocker medication (relative contraindication)

**Adverse Reactions:**
- hypotension
- congestive heart failure
- angina
- bradycardia
- headache
- nausea and vomiting
- dizziness

## NOTES ON ADMINISTRATION
**Routes of Administration:**
- IVP
- intravenous infusion
- oral

**Onset of Action:**
- IVP: immediate
- oral: 30–60 minutes

**Drug Interactions:**
- concomitant use of amiodarone, digoxin, and beta blockers may produce additive cardiac depression
- concomitant use of cimetidine may increase the bioavailability of diltiazem
- diltiazem may increase the bioavailability of carbamazepine, digoxin, and theophylline

**Adult Dosage:**

  *initial dose:*

  * 0.25 mg/kg IVP over 2 minutes

    40 kg = 10 mg (2.0 ml)

    60 kg = 15 mg (3.0 ml)

    80 kg = 20 mg (4.0 ml)

  *2nd dose (if necessary) after 15 minutes:*

  * 0.35 mg/kg IVP over 2 minutes

    40 kg = 14 mg (2.8 ml)

    60 kg = 21 mg (4.2 ml)

    80 kg = 28 mg (5.6 ml)

  *initial intravenous infusion:*

  * 5.0–10 mg/hour; dilute 100 mg (200 ml) in 100 ml of normal saline (1.0 mg/1.0 ml)

  *adjusted intravenous infusion:*

  * 15 mg/hour; dilute 150 mg (300 ml) in 150 ml of normal saline (1.0 mg/1.0 ml)

  *oral maintenance therapy:*

  * 120–360 mg per day (diltiazem is packaged in 30 mg tablets or 120 mg, 180 mg, or 240 mg CD capsules)

#### DOPAMINE

| | |
|---|---|
| **Generic Name:** | dopamine |
| **Trade Name:** | Intropin® |
| **Class:** | sympathomimetic |
| **Standard Supply:** | 400 mg/5.0 ml |
| | 400 mg in a 250 ml bag of D5W (1,600 µg/ml premixed solution) |

**Mechanism of Action:**

  * increases cardiac rate and contractility
  * causes peripheral vasoconstriction

**Dose-dependent Effects:**

- 1.0—2.0 µg/kg/minute: may dilate vessels in the kidneys and mesentery; may increase urine output; may decrease blood pressure
- 2.0–10 µg/kg/minute: increases heart rate and myocardial contractility
- 10–20 µg/kg/minute: causes peripheral vasoconstriction and hypertension

**Indications:**

- cardiogenic shock
- hemodynamically significant hypotension associated with CHF
- hemodynamically significant hypotension that is unresponsive to IV fluid resuscitation
- hemodynamically significant hypotension commensurate with the return of spontaneous pulses

**Contraindications:**

- hypovolemic shock
- pheochromocytoma (a tumor of the adrenal gland)

**Adverse Reactions:**

- arrhythmias
- tachycardia
- hypertension
- extravasation may cause tissue necrosis
- chest pain
- palpitations
- dyspnea
- headache
- nausea and vomiting

## NOTES ON ADMINISTRATION
**Route of Administration:**

- intravenous infusion

**Onset of Action:**

- immediate

**Drug Interaction:**

- this medication may be deactivated by sodium bicarbonate

**Adult Dosage:**

- 2.5–20 µg/kg/minute: initiate the infusion at 2.5 µg/kg/minute and titrate to effect
- if the patient's blood pressure is less than 70 mm Hg systolic, initiate the infusion at 5.0 µg/kg/minute
- if the patient's blood pressure is greater than 70 mm Hg systolic, initiate the infusion at 2.5 µg/kg/minute

### EPINEPHRINE

| | |
|---|---|
| **Generic Name:** | epinephrine |
| **Trade Name:** | Adrenalin® |
| **Class:** | catecholamine |
| **Standard Supply:** | • 1.0 mg/10 ml (1:10,000) |
| | • 1.0 mg/1.0 ml (1:1,000) |
| | • 30 mg/30 ml (1:1,000) |

**Mechanism of Action:**

- stimulates A-adrenergic receptors
- stimulates β-adrenergic ($\beta_1$ and $\beta_2$) receptors; β-adrenergic effects of epinephrine are more profound
- A-adrenergic effects
    1. arterial vasoconstriction
    2. increased systemic vascular resistance

- β₁-adrenergic effects
    1. increased heart rate
    2. increased cardiac automaticity
    3. increased cardiac contractility
    4. lowers the threshold for defibrillation
    5. may restore electrical activity in asystole
- β₂-adrenergic effects
    1. relaxes bronchial smooth muscle, resulting in bronchodilation

**Indications:**

- asthma
- reversible bronchospasm associated with COPD
- severe allergic reaction (anaphylaxis)
- hemodynamically significant bradycardia
- cardiac arrest
    1. ventricular fibrillation
    2. pulseless ventricular tachycardia
    3. asystole
    4. PEA

**Contraindications:**

- none in the emergency setting

**Adverse Reactions:**

- hypertension
- tachycardia
- anxiety
- nausea
- vomiting
- angina
- arrhythmias
- sweating
- palpitations

- headache
- tremors

## NOTES ON ADMINISTRATION

### Routes of Administration:

- IVP
- ET
- IM
- subcutaneous (SQ)
- intravenous infusion

### Onset of Action:

- immediate

### Drug Interactions:

- potentiates effects of other sympathomimetic drugs
- may be deactivated by sodium bicarbonate
- may not achieve desired effects in the presence of acidosis

### Adult Dosage:

- in cardiac arrest:
  1. 1.0 mg (1:10,000) IVP every 3–5 minutes or
  2. 2.0–2.5 mg (1:1,000) ET every 3–5 minutes
- for anaphylaxis, asthma, and reversible bronchospasm associated with COPD:
  1. 0.1–0.3 mg (1:1,000) SQ or IM
  2. 0.2–0.75 mg (1:10,000) ET or IVP if cardiovascular collapse occurs
- as a vasopressor agent: add 1.0 mg into a 250 mL bag of normal saline (4.0 µg/1.0 ml concentration) and infuse at 2.0–10 µg/minute (30–150 gtts/minute)

## EPTIFIBATIDE

| | |
|---|---|
| **Generic Name:** | eptifibatide |
| **Trade Names:** | Integrelin® |

| Classes: | antiplatelet agent, glycoprotein (GP) IIb/IIIa inhibitor |
| --- | --- |
| Standard Supply: | • 20 mg/10 ml vial |
| | • 75 mg/100 ml bottle (requires refrigeration) |

**Mechanism of Action:**

- reversibly binds with GP IIb/IIIa receptors on the surface of platelets, inhibiting platelet aggregation. (GP IIb/IIIa receptor blockade interferes with the binding of fibrinogen and other platelet aggregation modulators to the surface of platelets, thus preventing aggregation.)

**Indications:**

- acute coronary syndrome
- unstable angina
- PTCA or atherectomy
- reduce complications associated with PTCA
- non Q wave MI

**Contraindications:**

- active internal bleeding or recent history (within 30 days) of clinically significant gastrointestinal or genitourinary bleeding
- history of stroke with current residual neurological deficit, or within the past 2 years
- bleeding disorder, condition, or predisposition
- concomitant use of Coumadin® (warfarin), or use within the past 7 days unless prothrombin time is <1.2 times control
- thrombocytopenia (<100,000 cells/µl)
- trauma or major surgery within the past 6 weeks
- intracranial neoplasm
- arteriovenous malformation, aneurysm, or evidence of aortic dissection
- severe uncontrolled hypertension (systolic blood pressure >180 mm Hg/diastolic blood pressure >110 mm Hg)
- history of vasculitis

- concomitant use of another GP IIb/IIIa inhibitor
- acute pericarditis
- known hypersensitivity to eptifibatide

**Adverse Reactions:**

- bleeding (The most common sites of spontaneous bleeding include venous and arterial access sites. Major bleeding has been demonstrated to occur more often in patients who are >65 years old, <75 kg, with a history of gastrointestinal disease, and patients receiving thrombolytics or heparin.
- hemorrhagic stroke and intracranial bleeding
- thrombocytopenia

**NOTES ON ADMINISTRATION**

- Heparin should be concomitantly administered and monitored with eptifibatide.
- Due to the risk of spontaneous bleeding during administration of eptifibatide, the following procedures should be avoided whenever possible: arterial and venous punctures, intramuscular injection, placement of a urinary catheter, placement of a nasogastric tube, and nasotracheal intubation.

**Routes of Administration:**

- IVP
- intravenous infusion

**Onset of Action:**

- several minutes

**Drug Interactions:**

- other medications that affect hemostasis: thrombolytics, oral anticoagulants, aspirin and other nonsteroidal anti-inflammatory agents, dipyridamole, ticlopidine, and clopidogrel
- eptifibatide is not compatible in the same IV line with Lasix® (furosemide)
- herbal products containing ginkgo, biloba, ginger, and garlic

**Adult Dosage:**

*for acute coronary syndrome:*

· 180 µg/kg IVPush then
· 2.0 µg/kg/minute intravenous infusion for 72 hours, until discharge or if angioplasty or coronary artery bypass graft (CABG) procedure, then 20–24 hours post this procedure (IV pump required for intravenous infusion of eptibibatide)

*for percutaneous coronary intervention (PCI) in patients not presenting with an acute coronary syndrome:*

· 135 µg/kg IVP immediately before PTCA then
· 0.5 µg/kg/minute, continued for 20–24 hours

**Caveats:**

Weight-based dosing of eptifibatide and concomitant heparin essential to decrease the incidence of bleeding; infusion pump required for intravenous infusion administration of eptifibatide).

**FUROSEMIDE**

| | |
|---|---|
| **Generic Name:** | furosemide |
| **Trade Name:** | Lasix® |
| **Class:** | diuretic |
| **Standard Supply:** | · 40 mg/4.0 ml |
| | · 20 mg/2.0 ml |

**Mechanism of Action:**

· causes excretion of large volumes of urine within 5–30 minutes of administration
· inhibits sodium and chloride reabsorption in the kidney
· causes venous vasodilation

**Indications:**

· fluid overload in CHF
· pulmonary edema

**Contraindications:**

- hypovolemia
- hypotension
- pregnancy (furosemide has been known to cause fetal abnormalities)

**Adverse Reactions:**

- dehydration
- electrolyte disturbances
- hypotension
- arrhythmias
- nausea and vomiting

## NOTES ON ADMINISTRATION
**Route of Administration:**

- IVP

**Onset of Action:**

- 5 minutes

**Drug Interactions:**

- incompatible with diazepam, diphenhydramine, and thiamine
- lithium (may cause toxic levels of this medication)

**Adult Dosage:**

- 0.5–1.0 mg/kg (usually 20–40 mg) slow IVP
- A patient already taking prescribed furosemide may require a larger dose to achieve desired effects.

### LIDOCAINE HCL 2%

| | |
|---|---|
| **Generic Name:** | lidocaine HCL (2%) |
| **Trade Name:** | Xylocaine® |
| **Class:** | antiarrhythmic |

**Standard Supply:**          • 100 mg/5 ml

• 1 g/25 ml

• 2.0 g in a 250 ml bag of D$_5$W
(4.0 mg/ml premixed solution)

• 2.0 g in a 500 ml bag of D$_5$W
(4.0 mg/ml premixed solution)

**Mechanism of Action:**

• suppresses ventricular ectopy

• increases ventricular fibrillation threshold

**Indications:**

• ventricular fibrillation

• pulseless ventricular tachycardia

• stable ventricular tachycardia

• wide complex tachycardia of uncertain origin

• premature PVCs:

1. more than six PVCs per minute

2. two or more PVCs in a row

3. multiformed PVCs

4. R-on-T phenomenon

• post successful defibrillation from ventricular tachycardia or ventricular fibrillation

**Contraindications:**

• known hypersensitivity to the medication

• ventricular escape rhythm

• idioventricular rhythm

• usually in second-degree Mobitz II and complete (third-degree) heart block

• do not administer lidocaine to treat ventricular ectopy if the heart rate is less than 60 beats/minute

**Adverse Reactions:**

• central nervous system depression, including coma

• seizures

- hypotension
- drowsiness
- paraesthesia
- tremors
- heart blocks
- nausea and vomiting
- cardiac arrest

## NOTES ON ADMINISTRATION
### Routes of Administration:
- IVP
- intravenous infusion
- ET

### Onset of Action:
- 1–5 minutes

### Drug Interactions:
- none in the emergency setting

### Adult Dosage:
- rhythms with a pulse
    1. 1.0–1.5 mg/kg IVP
    2. additional IVP boluses: 0.5–0.75 mg/kg every 10 minutes to a total of 3.0 mg/kg
- rhythms without a pulse (ventricular fibrillation and pulseless ventricular tachycardia):
    1. 1.0–1.5 mg/kg IVP every 3–5 minutes to a total of 3.0 mg/kg
- following the return of pulses: 2.0–4.0 mg/minute intravenous infusion

For adult ET administration, deliver 2.0–2.5 times the recommended IVP dose and dilute with normal saline.

NOTE: The dosage may need to be decreased for the elderly patient as well as patients with liver disease.

## MAGNESIUM SULFATE

| | |
|---|---|
| **Generic Name:** | magnesium sulfate |
| **Trade Name:** | Magnesium Sulfate® |
| **Classes:** | electrolyte, anticonvulsant, antiarrhythmic |
| **Standard Supply:** | 1.0 g/2.0 ml |

**Mechanism of Action:**

- stabilizes muscle cell membranes by interacting with the sodium/potassium exchange system
- alters calcium's effect on myocardial conduction
- depresses the central nervous system
- causes smooth muscle relaxation

**Indications:**

- obstetrical
  1. pregnancy-induced hypertension
  2. seizures associated with preeclampsia
  3. preterm labor
- cardiac arrhythmias
  1. Torsades de Pointes
  2. ventricular fibrillation/pulseless ventricular tachycardia

  There is growing support in advanced cardiac life support for use of magnesium sulfate as a first-line agent in the treatment of myocardial ischemia, MI and cardiac arrhythmias.

**Contraindications:**

- heart blocks
- respiratory depression
- kidney failure

**Adverse Reactions:**

- hypotension
- respiratory depression or arrest

- cardiac arrest
- hypotension
- drowsiness
- arrhythmias

NOTE: Calcium chloride should be administered as an antidote to magnesium sulfate if respiratory depression occurs.

## NOTES ON ADMINISTRATION

### Routes of Administration:

- IVP
- IM
- intravenous infusion

### Onset of Action:

- immediate

### Drug Interactions:

- none in the emergency setting

### Adult Dosage:

- for seizures associated with preeclampsia:
  1. 3.0—6.0 g IVP or infusion delivered over 10–15 minutes
  2. repeat bolus 2.0–4.0 g IVP or infusion over 10–15 minutes
  3. if intravenous access cannot be established: 2.0–4.0 g IM

  Because of the volume of this medication, the IM dose should be divided in half and administered IM at separate sites (usually each gluteus). An infusion may be prepared by adding the medication to a 50 ml or 100 ml bag of normal saline.

- for preterm labor:
  1. 4.0–6.0 g IVP or infusion delivered over 10–15 minutes
  2. follow initial bolus with 2.0 g/hour infusion, which may be continued until uterine contractions are reduced to one or less every 10 minutes

- for cardiac arrhythmias:
  1. 1.0–2.0 g IVP or infusion delivered over 1–2 minutes
- for torsade de pointes:
  1. 1.0–2.0 g IVP or infusion delivered over 1–2 minutes
  2. follow initial bolus with 1.0–2.0 g infusion delivered over 1 hour

## MORPHINE SULFATE

| | |
|---|---|
| **Generic Name:** | morphine sulfate |
| **Trade Name:** | Morphine Sulfate® |
| **Class:** | narcotic analgesic |
| **Standard Supply:** | 10 mg/1.0 ml |

**Mechanism of Action:**

- provides relief of pain
- causes central nervous system depression
- causes peripheral venous dilation (↓preload)
- decreases systemic vascular resistance (↓afterload)

**Indications:**

- chest pain in MI
- pain associated with burns
- pain associated with musculoskeletal injuries
- pain associated with kidney stones
- pulmonary edema

**Contraindications:**

- known hypersensitivity to the medication
- acute bronchospasm or asthma
- respiratory depression
- head injury
- abdominal pain of unknown etiology
- hypotension

**Adverse Reactions:**
- central nervous system depression
- hypotension
- nausea and vomiting
- respiratory depression
- respiratory arrest
- constricted pupils

## NOTES ON ADMINISTRATION

**Routes of Administration:**
- IVP
- IM

**Onset of Action:**
- immediate

**Drug Interactions:**
- central nervous system and respiratory depression can occur when administered with antihistamines, sedatives, hypnotics, barbiturates, antidepressants, and alcohol
- effects of this medication can be reversed by administration of naloxone (Narcan)

**Adult Dosage:**
- for relief of pain: 2.0–10 mg slow IVP or IM
- for cardiogenic chest pain: 1.0–3.0 mg IV
  Additional doses of 2.0 mg every 2–10 minutes may be administered to titrate for relief of pain.
- for pulmonary edema: 1.0–3.0 mg IVP or according to protocol

## NITROGLYCERIN

| | |
|---|---|
| **Generic Name:** | nitroglycerin |
| **Trade Names:** | Nitrostat®, Nitro-Bid® |
| **Classes:** | vasodilator, antianginal |

**Standard Supply:**         0.4 mg tablet

**Mechanism of Action:**

- relaxes vascular smooth muscle resulting in
    1. coronary artery vasodilation
    2. relief of chest pain by dilating coronary arteries
    3. decreased return of blood to the heart (preload)
    4. decreased myocardial oxygen demand
    5. decreased workload on the heart
    6. decreased systemic vascular resistance (afterload)

**Indications:**

- signs and symptoms associated with angina pectoris
- signs and symptoms associated with MI
- congestive heart failure with pulmonary edema

**Contraindications:**

- the patient already has taken the maximum prescribed dose of the medication
- hypotension
- shock
- head injury

**Adverse Reactions:**

- hypotension
- headache
- dizziness
- bradycardia
- weakness
- fainting
- tachycardia
- flushing and feelings of warmth
- nausea and vomiting
- bitter taste
- burning or tingling sensations in the mouth

## NOTES ON ADMINISTRATION
**Route of Administration:**

- sublingual (SL)

**Onset of Action:**

- immediate

**Drug Interactions:**

- increased effects with other vasodilators
- alcohol (may cause severe hypotension)
- beta-adrenergic blockers (may cause orthostatic hypotension)
- Viagra (concomitant use may cause severe hypotension)

**Adult Dosage:**

- 0.4 mg SL
- 0.4 mg SL may be repeated after 5 minutes, and then again after 5 more minutes, for a total of 3 doses (1.2 mg)

**Caveat:**

Nitroglycerin must be protected from light and expires quickly once the bottle has been opened.

### OXYGEN

| | |
|---|---|
| **Generic Name:** | oxygen |
| **Trade Name:** | Oxygen® |
| **Class:** | natural gas |

There is 21% oxygen present in atmospheric air. Arterial partial pressure is represented by the abbreviation *Pa*. The normal arterial partial pressure for oxygen ($PaO_2$) = 100 torr (range = 80–100 torr).

**Standard Supply:**

- Oxygen is stored in steel-green or aluminum gray cylinders under pressure of 2,000–2,200 psi.
- Oxygen cylinders are designated by letters to identify their size. D, E, and M cylinders are the most common in emergency care.

- Oxygen flow from a cylinder is controlled by a regulator that reduces high pressure and controls liter flow.

**Mechanism of Action:**

- rapidly diffuses across the alveolar walls and binds to hemoglobin in the red blood cells
- reverses deleterious effects of hypoxemia on the brain, heart, and other tissues in the body
- increases arterial oxygen tension ($PaO_2$)
- increases hemoglobin saturation
- is necessary for the efficient breakdown of glucose into a usable energy: adenosine triphosphate (ATP)

This process is known as *aerobic metabolism*, metabolism that occurs in the presence of oxygen.

**Indications:**

- any condition in which systemic or local hypoxemia may be present, including
  1. dyspnea or respiratory arrest from any cause
  2. chest pain
  3. shock
  4. cardiopulmonary arrest
  5. unconsciousness
  6. any submersion accident
  7. toxic inhalations
  8. stroke
  9. head injury
  10. seizures
  11. any critical patient, including all forms of trauma and medical emergencies

**Contraindications:**

- none in the emergency setting
- There is concern that patients with COPD may experience respiratory depression with the administration of

high flow oxygen. COPD patients' respiration tends to be regulated by a *hypoxic drive* in which respiration is stimulated by the brain's perception of a low oxygen level, rather than by a high carbon dioxide level, as in normal patients. High flow oxygen administration to the COPD patient does not have a clinically significant effect on respiration if used for a brief time in an emergency setting.

**Adverse Reactions:**

- none in the emergency setting

## NOTES ON ADMINISTRATION

**Routes of Administration:**

- inhalation
    1. nasal cannula
    2. simple face mask
    3. nonrebreather mask
- ventilation
    1. any ventilatory device, for example, bag-valve-mask (BVM), automatic transport ventilator (ATV), or pocket mask with oxygen inlet

**Onset of Action:**

- variable

**Drug Interaction:**

- none in the emergency setting

**Oxygen Delivery Devices:**

| Device | Flow Rate | % of $O_2$ Delivered |
| --- | --- | --- |
| nasal cannula | 1–6 l/minute | 24–44% |
| simple face mask | 8–10 l/minute | 35–60% |
| nonrebreather mask | 15 l/minute | 95% |

**Caveat:**

NOTE: Other oxygen delivery systems include the pocket mask, BVM, flow-restricted oxygen-powered ventilation device, and ATV.

## SODIUM BICARBONATE

| | |
|---|---|
| **Generic Name:** | sodium bicarbonate |
| **Trade Name:** | Sodium Bicarbonate® |
| **Class:** | alkalinizing agent |
| **Standard Supply:** | 50 mEq/50 ml |

**Mechanism of Action:**

- increases pH (alkalinization) in the blood and urine
- acts as buffering (neutralizing) agent for acids in the blood and interstitial fluid
- increases tricyclic antidepressant excretion from the body in an overdose setting (by making the urine more alkaline)

**Indications:**

- severe acidosis refractory to ventilation
- tricyclic antidepressant overdose
- documented metabolic acidosis
- considered after 10 minutes in resuscitation of cardiac arrest

NOTE: Ventilatory management, prompt defibrillation, and the administration of epinephrine and lidocaine should always proceed use of sodium bicarbonate.

**Contraindications:**

- none in the emergency setting

**Adverse Reactions:**

- paradoxical intracellular acidosis
- metabolic alkalosis

NOTE: Sodium bicarbonate transiently raises arterial $PCO_2$. Administration of this medication must be accompanied by efficient ventilation to blow off excess carbon dioxide.

## NOTES ON ADMINISTRATION
### Route of Administration:
- IVP

### Onset of Action:
- immediate

### Interactions:
- inactivates sympathomimetic medications (e.g., epinephrine, dopamine, and isoproterenol when they come in contact, i.e., when given together)
- may produce a chalky precipitate of calcium carbonate when administered together with calcium chloride, calcium gluconate, atropine, morphine sulfate, aminophylline, and magnesium

### Adult Dosage:
- 1.0 mEq/kg IVP
- repeat every 10 minutes: 0.5 mEq/kg

### TIROFIBAN

| | |
|---|---|
| **Generic Name:** | tirofiban |
| **Trade Names:** | Aggrastat® |
| **Classes:** | antiplatelet agent, GP IIb/IIIa inhibitor |
| **Standard Supply:** | 250 µg/ml in 50 ml vial |
| | premixed 50 µg/ml in 500 ml D5W or normal saline |

### Mechanism of Action:
- reversibly binds with GP IIb/IIIa receptors on the surface of platelets, inhibiting platelet aggregation (GP IIb/IIIa receptor blockade interferes with the binding of

fibrinogen and other platelet aggregation modulators to the surface of platelets, thus preventing aggregation.)

**Indications:**

- acute coronary syndrome
- PTCA or arteriectomy, includes intravenous infusion monitoring during prehospital interfacility transportation
- unstable angina
- AMI

**Contraindications:**

- active internal bleeding or recent history (within 30 days) of clinically significant gastrointestinal or genitourinary bleeding
- history of stroke with current residual neurological deficit, or within the past 2 years
- bleeding disorder, condition, or predisposition
- concomitant use of Coumadin® (warfarin), or use within the past 7 days unless prothrombin time is <1.2 times control
- thrombocytopenia (<100,000 cells/µl)
- trauma or major surgery within the past 6 weeks
- intracranial neoplasm
- arteriovenous malformation, aneurysm, or evidence of aortic dissection
- severe uncontrolled hypertension (systolic blood pressure >180 mm Hg/diastolic blood pressure >110 mm Hg)
- history of vasculitis
- concomitant use of another GP IIb/IIIa inhibitor
- acute pericarditis
- known hypersensitivity to tirofiban

**Adverse Reactions:**

- bleeding (The most common sites of spontaneous bleeding include venous and arterial access sites. Major bleeding has been demonstrated to occur more often in patients who are >65 years old, <75 kg, with a history of gastrointestinal disease, and patients receiving thrombolytics or heparin.)

- fever, chills, diaphoresis, and dizziness
- hemorrhagic stroke and intracranial bleeding
- sinus bradycardia
- thrombocytopenia

## NOTES ON ADMINISTRATION

- Heparin should be concomitantly administered and monitored with tirofiban.
- Due to the risk of spontaneous bleeding during administration of tirofiban, the following procedures should be avoided whenever possible: arterial and venous punctures, intramuscular injection, placement of a urinary catheter, placement of a nasogastric tube and nasotracheal intubation.

**Route of Administration:**

- IVP
- intravenous infusion

**Onset of Action:**

- several minutes

**Drug Interactions:**

- medications that affect hemostasis: thrombolytics, oral anticoagulants, aspirin and other nonsteroidal anti-inflammatory drugs (NSAIDs), dipyridamole, ticlopidine, and copidogrel
- herbal products containing ginkgo, biloba, ginger, and garlic

**Adult Dosage:**

- 0.4 µg/kg/minute IVP for 30 minutes then
- 0.1 µg/kg/minute intravenous infusion, for a minimum of 48 hours and 12–24 hours post angioplasty

**Caveat:**

Weight-based dosing of tirofiban and concomitant heparin is essential to decrease the incidence of bleeding. An infusion pump is required for intravenous infusion administration of tirofiban.

### VERAPAMIL HCL

| | |
|---|---|
| **Generic Name:** | verapamil HCl |
| **Trade Names:** | Calan®, Isoptin® |
| **Class:** | calcium-channel blocker |
| **Standard Supply:** | 5.0 mg/2.0 ml |

**Mechanism of Action:**
- causes vascular dilation
- selectively inhibits slow calcium channels in cardiac tissue
- slows conduction through the AV node
- inhibits reentry during PSVT
- decreases the rate of ventricular response associated with atrial fibrillation and atrial flutter
- reduces myocardial oxygen demand
- causes coronary artery vasodilation
- causes peripheral vasodilation

**Indications:**
- narrow-complex PSVT refractory to administration of adenosine
- atrial fibrillation with rapid ventricular response
- atrial flutter with rapid ventricular response

**Contraindications:**
- hypotension
- cardiogenic shock
- wide complex tachycardia

- ventricular tachycardia
- WPW syndrome
- sick-sinus syndrome
- beta-blocker medications

**Adverse Reactions:**

- bradycardia
- hypotension
- headache
- dizziness
- heart block
- congestive heart failure with pulmonary edema
- nausea and vomiting
- asystole

## NOTES ON ADMINISTRATION

### Route of Administration:

- slow IVP (over 1–2 minutes)

### Onset of Action:

- 1–10 minutes

### Drug Interactions:

- beta-blocker medications
- calcium chloride may be administered to prevent hypotensive effects in the management of a calcium-channel blocker overdose

### Adult Dosage:

- 2.5–5.0 mg slow IVP
- repeat in 15–30 minutes: 5.0–10 mg IVP up to a maximum of 30 mg in 30 minutesπ

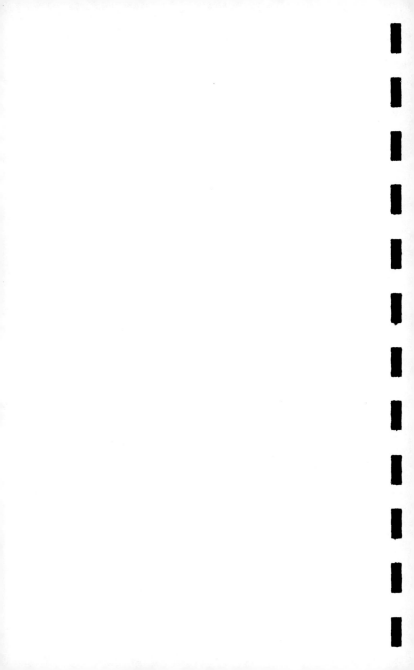

# Appendix B
## Emergency Cardiac Care Guidelines

••••••••••••••••••••••••••••••••••••••••••••••••••••••••••••••••••••••••

The following tables include the Emergency Cardiac Care Guidelines based on the American Heart Association's 1997–1999 *Handbook of Emergency Cardiovascular Care for Health Care Providers*. These are guidelines for possible interventions for the patient who presents with cardiac compromise. Regardless of the clinical setting, the provider must be aware of protocols and guidelines that affect and govern treatment modalities. Now, more than ever, changes in treatment, drugs, and drug dosages occur frequently.

This appendix is not meant to be prescriptive, merely a baseline for assessment and a memory-jogger for the more common approaches to patient care. It is the responsibility of the provider to maintain commitment to current knowledge and implementation of patient care standards in a specific work environment.

## ADVANCED CARDIAC LIFE
## SUPPORT ALGORITHMS

### Ventricular Fibrillation and
### Pulseless Ventricular Tachycardia

• ABCs
• Perform CPR until defibrillator available
• VF/VT present on defibrillator
↓

Defibrillate up to 3 times if needed for
VF/VT at 200J, 200-300J, 360J
↓

Persistent or recurrent VF/VT ?
↓

CPR if no pulse
Intubate at once
Establish IV access (at least 16 G)
↓

Epinephrine 1:10,000 **1.0 mg q 3–5 min** IVPush
↓

• Defibrillate with up to 360 J* within
30–60 seconds after dose of medication
↓

Lidocaine **1.5 mg/kg IVPush q 3–5 min** to a
total dose of 3 mg/kg 4
↓

Consider amiodarone
↓

Bretylium 5 mg/kg IVP. Repeat in 5 minutes at 10 mg/kg
(Consider Bicarb 1 mEq/kg)
↓

Defibrillate 360 J, 30–60 seconds after
each dose of medication
(Consider magnesium sulfate for refractory VF)

*May use stacked shocks of 200J, 200–300J, 360J.

## Asystole

- Confirm asystole in 2 leads
- Continue CPR
- Intubate at once
- Obtain IV access

↓

Consider possible causes
Hypoxia, Hyperkalemia, Hypokalemia,
Hypothermia, Acidosis, OD

↓

Consider Immediate Transcutaneous
Pacing (TCP)

↓

Epinephrine 1:10,000 **1.0 mg q 3–5 min** IVP

↓

Atropine **1 mg IVPush, repeat every 3–5 min**
up to a total of 0.04 mg/kg

↓

May consider Bicarb 1 mEq/kg
with consideration to
patient's clinical situation

↓

Consider termination of efforts
per local protocol and policy

## Pulseless Electrical Activity (PEA)

*PEA includes:*
EMD, pseudo-EMD, idioventricular,
ventricular escape rhythms,
bradyasystolic rhythms
↓
• Continue CPR
• Intubate at once
• Obtain IV access
↓
Consider Possible Causes
**P**ulmonary Embolism, **A**cidosis, **T**ension
Pneumothorax, **C**ardiac Tamponade,
**H**ypovolemia, **H**ypoxia, **H**ypothermia,
**H**yperkalemia, **M**I, **D**rug Overdose
↓
Epinephrine 1:10,000 **1.0 mg q 3–5 min** IVPush
↓
Consider 250 ml fluid bolus
↓
If absolute bradycardia (HR <60)
or relative bradycardia, give
Atropine **1 mg IVPush q 3–5 min** up to
a total of 0.04 mg/kg
Consider Immediate Transcutaneous
Pacing (TCP)

---

**NOTE:** When preparing for synchronized cardioversion, premedicate the patient whenever possible. Some possible choices might include diazapam or morphine sulfate. This will be a clinical based on patient presentation and urgency of the situation.

## Sustained Ventricular Tachycardia With a Pulse

### Stable: Heart rate < 150 without compromise

- Assess ABCs
- High-flow oxygen
- Obtain IV access
- Attach to monitor and assess vital signs

↓

Lidocaine **1–1.5 mg/kg IVPush**
Rebolus at 0.5–0.75 mg/kg IVPush Every 5–10 min until
V-tach resolves, or until a total dose of 3 mg/kg is given

↓

Procainamide 20–30 mg/min, max total
17 mg/kg

↓

Consider amiodarone

↓

Bretylium 5–10 mg/kg over 8–10 min, to a
max of 30 mg/kg total dose

↓

**Synchronized cardioversion
100J, 200J, 300J, 360J**

### Unstable: HR > 150 and Compromised

ABCs, O₂, IV
Consider brief trial of medications

↓

**Unsynchronized Cardioversion** if patient is
unconscious, hypotensive, or presents with
pulmonary edema. May **attempt** synch
cardioversion with sedation, but not to
delay therapy.
**100J, 200J, 300J, 360J**

## Wide-Complex Tachycardia of Uncertain Type

**If patient is unstable (HR > 150) now or becomes
unstable—perform
Synchronized cardioversion at 100 J,
200 J, 300 J, 360 J**
↓
**STABLE:**
Assess ABCs, high-flow oxygen,
obtain IV access, assess vital signs
↓
Lidocaine 1–1.5 mg/kg IVPush,
may rebolus at 0.5–0.75 mg/kg IVPush to a total
of 3 mg/kg
↓
Adenosine 6 mg, rapid IVPush over 1–3 seconds,
if no response in 1–2 minutes, then
↓
Adenosine 12 mg, rapid IVPush over 1–3 seconds,
may repeat once in 1–2 minutes
↓
Procainamide 20-30 mg/min, max total
17 mg/kg
↓
Bretylium 5–10 mg/kg over 8–10 minutes,
maximum total 30 mg/kg
↓
**Synchronized cardioversion
100J, 200J, 300 J, 360J**

## Bradycardia
## (HR < 60 beats/minute)

- Assess ABCs, secure airway
- High-flow oxygen
- Obtain IV access
- Attach monitor and assess vital signs

↓

**Rate too slow?**

↓

**Serious signs and symptoms?**

↓

**NO sign/symptoms**

↓

If patient presents with Type II second-degree
or third-degree AV block, be ready to use
transcutaneous external pacing (TCP).
If delayed or unavailable, give **Atropine
0.5-1.0 mg IVPq 3–5 min
to a total dose of 0.03–0.04 mg/kg**


**YES signs/symptoms**
**Atropine 0.5–1.0 mg IVPush,** may repeat
every 3–5 minutes up to a total of
0.03–0.04  mg/kg
(May use up to 3 mg total for
severe cases)

↓

Transcutaneous  Pacing (TCP)

↓

Dopamine 5-20 µg/kg/min
(For **BP < 70** start at 5 µg/kg/min and
for **BP > 70** start at 2.5 µg/kg/min)

↓

Epinephrine infusion 2–10  µg/min

## Supraventricular Tachycardia

### Unstable: (HR > 150)

ABCs, $O_2$, IV
↓
**Prepare for synchronized cardioversion
(consider sedation)**
• Synchronized cardioversion at 50 J,
100 J, 200 J, 300 J, & 360 J
↓
Reassess

### Stable:
Vagal maneuvers
↓
Adenosine **6 mg, rapid IVP over 1–3 seconds**
If no response, may give a bolus of
12 mg, rapid IVPush over 1–3 sec
May repeat 12 mg bolus in 1–2 minutes
↓
• **Consider complex width:**
NARROW COMPLEX → Normal or ↑ BP
Verapamil 2.5–5 mg IVPush
Verapamil 5–10 mg IVPush (in 15–30 minutes)

NARROW COMPLEX → Low or Unstable BP
Synchronized cardioversion

WIDE COMPLEX
Lidocaine 1–1.5 mg/kg IVPush
Procainamide 20–30 mg/min, maximum total
17 mg/kg
Synchronized cardioversion

## Atrial Fibrillation and Atrial Flutter

Assess ABCs, high-flow $O_2$, obtain IV access, attach monitor, and assess vital signs
↓
Unstable—synchronized cardioversion at
100 J,  200 J, 300 J, 360 J*

Stable → Consider use of the following:
Diltiazem, β-Blockers, Verapamil, Digoxin, Procainamide, Quinidine, Anticoagulants

*In cases of **atrial flutter** and **PSVT**, the energy required for synchronized cardioversion begins with 50 J.

## Polymorphic Ventricular Tachycardia

ABCs, $O_2$, IV
↓
**Electrical** treatment of choice is unsynchronized
cardioversion in sustained tachycardia
Transcutaneous (overdrive) pacing
↓
**Magnesium Sulfate 1–2 g over**
1–2 minutes, followed by the same amount
infused over 1 hour

**UNSTABLE:**
Assess ABCs
↓
$O_2$, IV access
↓
Unsynchronized cardioversion at 200 J
200–300 J,  360 J
↓
If the patient becomes pulseless,
treat as ventricular fibrillation.

## Shock, Hypotension, and Pulmonary Edema

• Assess ABCs, high-flow $O_2$, obtain IV access, attach
monitor, and assess vital signs

↓

### WHAT IS THE NATURE OF THE PROBLEM?

**RATE:**      Go to the tachycardia or bradycardia algorithm

**VOLUME:**    Administer fluids, cause-specific interventions,
consider vasopressors, AND

↓

**PUMP:**      **WHAT IS THE BLOOD PRESSURE?**

↓

| Systolic BP < 70 | Systolic BP 70–100 | Diastolic BP > 110 |
|---|---|---|
| 1. 250–500 ml Fluid Challenge | 1. Dopamine | 1. Nitroglycerin (10–20 μg/min) |
| 2. Norepinephrine (0–5–30 μg/min) | | 2. Nitroprusside (0.1–5.0 μg/kg/min) |
| 3. Dopamine (5–20 μg/kg/min) | | |

Systolic BP > 100
1. Dobutamine (2–20 μg/kg/min)

↓

Consider other actions, especially for patients
in pulmonary edema.

↓

| **First Line:** | Lasix IV 0.5–1.0 mg/kg | Morphine IV 1–3 mg |
|---|---|---|
| | Nitroglycerin SL | Oxygen/Intubate PRN |
| **Second Line:** | Nitroglycerin IV (if BP > 100) | |
| | Nitroprusside IV (if BP > 100) | |
| | Dopamine IV (if BP < 100) | |
| | Dobutamine IV (if BP > 100) | |
| | PEEP, CPAP | |
| **Third Line:** | Thrombolytics & Lanoxin | |

## Acute Myocardial Infarction

Community emphasis on "Call First/Call Fast, Call 911"
↓
• **EMS system**
Oxygen-IV-cardiac monitor (1 2-Lead)-vital signs

• **Nitroglycerin**
Pain relief with narcotics
Notification of emergency center
Rapid transportation and prehospital screening for
thrombolytic therapy
Initiation of thrombolytic therapy
↓
• **Emergency center**
"Door-to-Drug" team protocol approach with rapid triage of
patients with chest pain and clinical decision maker established
(emergency physician, cardiologist, etc.)
↓
**Time interval in emergency center not to exceed 30–60 minutes to
receive thrombolytic therapy**
↓

| *Assessment Immediate:* | *Treatments to consider if there is evidence of coronary thrombosis:* |
|---|---|
| Vital signs | High-flow oxygen |
| Oxygen saturation | Nitroglycerin-SL, BP > 90 |
| Start IV | Morphine IV |
| 12-lead ECG | Aspirin PO |
| Brief history/physical | Thrombolytic Agents |
| Decide on eligibility for | Nitroglycerin IV |
| thrombolytic therapy | β-Blockers |
| *As soon as possible:* | Heparin IV |
| Chest X-ray | PTCA |
| Blood studies | Glycoprotein IIb/IIIa inhibitors |
| Consult | |

# Appendix C
# Quick Review of Assessment and Interventions for Patients and Arrhythmias

**APPROACH TO PATIENTS**

Once attention to ABCs and oxygen therapy has begun, securing an IV for possible administration of fluids and medications is usually the next step. Assessing and documenting vital signs and initial ECG analysis should follow. Remember dialogue with the patient, friends, and significant others is important.

In cases where more than one advanced life support (ALS) provider is present, there is almost simultaneous assessment, history taking, noting of the physical environment, and detailed physical examination. Questions should be appropriate to assess the chief complaint, history of present illness, medical history, any medication history, and allergies that may contribute to patient care decisions.

The patient's statements describing signs and symptoms are documented in the patient's own words. Clinical assessment, vital signs, and reassessment are done after each intervention. For example, if the patient received pain medication, the reassessment would include the patient presentation, vital signs, effect on the ECG rhythm, and the effect on the ectopics if applicable.

Following are guidelines for possible interventions for the patient who presents with cardiac compromise. Regardless of the clinical setting, the provider must be aware of protocols and guidelines that affect and govern treatment modalities. Changes in treatment often occur as a result of aggressive world wide investigations in the area of cardiovascular disease.

This section is not meant to be prescriptive, merely a baseline for assessment and a memory-jogger for the more common approaches to patient care. It is the responsibility of the provider to maintain commitment to the current knowledge and implementation of patient care standards in a specific work environment.

### For Slow Rates in Hypotensive and Hypoperfusing Patients

**Narrow QRS:** *Consider*
Atropine for rate
Dopamine for perfusion
Pacemaker
Epi infusion (clinical)

**Wide QRS:** *Consider*
Pacemaker
Dopamine for perfusion
Pacemaker
Epi infusion (clinical)

**AV Block with narrow QRS and rapid sinus rate:** *Consider*
Dopamine for perfusion
Pacemaker
Epi infusion

### For Ventricular Fibrillation

**Confirm "no pulse"**
Goal: To depolarize the
fibrillating myocardium

Defibrillation beginning at 200 J

Epinephrine
Lidocaine
Amiodarone

Bretylium
Magnesium

## For the Narrow QRS Tachycardia

**Stable:**
Goal: To slow down AV conduction and
provide a better perfusing ventricular rate
*Consider*
Vagal Maneuvers
Adenosine
Verapamil (first line for A-fib)

**Unstable:**
Patient is hypotensive and hypoperfusing

Goal: To depolarize the ectopic tachycardia

Synch CV beginning at 50 J
A-fib at 100 J

## For Asystole

**Confirmed in a another lead**
Goal: To maintain the patient and try to
support an underlying escape rhythm

CPR, Intubation
Epinephrine
Atropine
Pace
Consider causes

### DO NOT DEFIBRILLATE!

## For the Wide QRS Tachycardia

**VT stable:**
Goal: To make the irritable ventricular cells more refractory

*Consider*
Lidocaine
Bretylium or Procainamide

**VT unstable:**
Patient is hypotensive and hypoperfusing
Sync CV beginning at 100 J

**VT torsade**
Defibrillation beginning at 200 J

**VT pulseless**
Defibrillation beginning at 200 J

## For Pulseless Electrical Activity

**Identify the rhythm**

Goal: To identify any mechanical impairment to pulse and cardiac output

CPR (assess for pulses; ? MI tamponade/rupture)
Intubate (assess breath sounds; ? pneumothorax) IVs (fluid challenge; ? hypovolemia)
Epinephrine IV/ET
Atropine if there is a bradycardia

As you treat, reassess; assessment contributes to determining the cause.

## Grid for Assessing the Narrow QRS

Look at the P waves:

S →      1 (+) P for each QRS

J →      (−) P for each QRS or none

A →  $\begin{cases} \text{Tachy = regular} \\ \text{Flutter = flutter waves you can count} \\ \text{Fib = junk—no identifiable Ps, QRS irregular} \end{cases}$

## Analyzing the Narrow QRS Complex

### Sinus Rhythm (+)P plus QRS

60–100  = rhythm

<60     = bradycardia

>100    = tachycardia

irreg   = arrhythmia

SA block missed QRS

SA arrest misses >one QRS

### Junctional (−)P or none

40–60/minute   = junctional rhythm

60–100/minute = accelerated junction rhythm

>100/minute    = junctional tachycardia

### Atrial

Flutter waves between QRS complex   = atrial flutter

Irregular, chaotic baseline             = atrial fibrillation

Persistent, regular rate > 100/minute  = atrial tachycardia

### Premature P waves

(−) or absent                      = junctional

(+) premature P wave plus QRS = PAC

(+) premature P, no QRS          = blocked PAC

## Analyzing the Wide Complex QRS

### Ventricular

QRS different than underlying rhythm

QRS (+) and T wave (−)

QRS (−) and T wave (+)

Sinus P wave plot through the event

| | |
|---|---|
| 20–40/minute | = idioventricular rhythm |
| 40–100/minute | = accelerated ventricular rhythm |
| >100/minute | = ventricular tachycardia |
| >3 in a row | = ventricular tachycardia |
| Chaotic baseline | = ventricular fibrillation |

### Aberrant Ventricular Conduction

QRS premature

QRS different than underlying rhythm

QRS and T wave (+)

QRS (+) and T wave (−) (rare)

QRS preceded by PAC

### Torsade

Spindle-like effect

QRS rapid and (+) followed by QRS rapid and (−)

### PVCs

| | |
|---|---|
| Uniform | = similar in appearance |
| Multiform | = vary in appearance |
| Bigeminy | = every other beat is a PVC |
| Paired | = two PVCs in succession |
| Interpolated | = sandwiched between two normal QRS complexes |
| End-diastolic | = after a regularly anticipated P wave |
| R-on-T | = appears on any part of the preceding T wave |

**How to Assess a Monitor Pattern**

1. Is the rhythm supraventricular or ventricular in origin?
   a. If the QRS ≤0.10 second: it is likely supraventricular in origin.
   a. If the QRS >0.12 second: may be ventricular in origin.
2. If the QRS in 0.10 second or less: look to the left of the QRS. If there is a P for every QRS and it is
   a. (+), regular and consistent: it is probably sinus in origin.
   b. (−) or absent and the QRS rhythm is regular: it is probably junctional.
3. Is the PR interval ≤0.20 second and consistent?
   a. >0.20 second: consider AV conduction defect.
   b. Progressive prolongation of the PR interval (segment): consider AV conduction defect.
   c. No consistent PR interval and P wave rate different than ventricular rate: consider complete AV block.
4. Analyze if *different* QRS complexes are premature or escape. Plot out the P waves:
   a. If P waves plot out regularly: the ectopic is probably ventricular in origin, regardless of its looks.
   b. If P waves do not plot out regularly: the ectopic is probably supraventricular in origin, most likely atrial.
5. Calculate the rate:
   a. Plot P to P and QRS to QRS at the baseline, NOT peak to peak.
   b. If Ps and/or QRSs are regular: divide the number of large boxes between two regularly occurring wave forms and divide into 300.
   c. In rapid rates: divide the number of small boxes between two regularly occurring wave forms and divide into 1,500.
   d. For irregular rhythms, calculate the widest and narrowest R-R for the accurate rate range.

6. Describe any other deviation including:
   a. ST segment elevation or depression.
   b. T wave changes such as inversion or in appearance.
   c. QRS notching.
   d. Change rhythm.

## How to Look at a Monitor Pattern Using the 12-Lead ECG

1. What is the standard? This is the measurement against which we compare the amplitude of the wave forms.
2. What is the underlying rhythm?
3. Look for the acute changes, according to the surfaces of the heart: Qs, ST segment changes, T-wave inversion:
   a. Leads II, III, aVF: the inferior wall
   b. Leads I, aVL, $V_6$: left lateral wall
   c. $V_1 \rightarrow V_4$: anterior walls
   d. $V_{3R} \rightarrow$ right anterior wall
4. Look for ventricular conduction disturbances:
   a. Leads II, III, aVF: left anterior fascicle
   b. Leads I, aVL, $V_6$: left posterior fascicle
   c. Lead $V_1$ for RBBB
5. What is the axis?
6. What can happen next? Which lead to observe?

## List of Abbreviations

**ECG:**

| | |
|---|---|
| (+) | positive (as with deflections) |
| (−) | negative (as with deflections) |
| A-fib | atrial fibrillation |
| AIVR | accelerated idioventricular rhythm |
| AJR | accelerated junctional rhythm |
| AV | atrioventricular |
| AVNR | AV nodal reentry |

| | |
|---|---|
| CLBBB | complete left bundle branch block |
| IVR | idioventricular rhythm |
| LAD | left axis deviation |
| LAH | left anterior hemiblock |
| LBBB | left bundle branch block |
| LGL | Lown Ganong Levine (syndrome) |
| LPH | left posterior hemiblock, aka left posterior fascicular |
| M/F | multiformed (as with PVCs) |
| P′ | Pprime |
| PAC | premature atrial complex |
| PAT | paroxysmal atrial tachycardia |
| PJC | premature junctional complex |
| PR | P-R interval (intrinsic) |
| PSVT | paroxysmal supraventricular tachycardia |
| PVC | premature ventricular complex |
| RAD | right axis deviation |
| RBBB | right bundle branch block |
| SA | sino-atrial node, aka sinus node |
| SVT | supraventricular tachycardia |
| TdP | torsade de pointes |
| U/F | uniform (as with PVCs) |
| UTD | unable to determine |
| VAT | ventricular activation time |
| VF | ventricular fibrillation |
| VT | ventricular tachycardia |
| WPW | Wolff Parkinson White (syndrome) |

**Anatomy and Physiology**

| | |
|---|---|
| ATP | adenosine triphosphate |
| Ca++ | calcium (electrolyte) |
| CABG | coronary artery bypass graft |
| CFX | circumflex (coronary artery) |
| GI | gastrointestinal |
| K+ | potassium (electrolyte) |
| LAD | left anterior descending (coronary artery) |
| LAE | left atrial enlargement |

| LAF | left anterior fascicle |
| LCA | left coronary artery |
| LPF | left posterior fascicle |
| LVH | left ventricular hypertrophy |
| MI | myocardial infarction |
| Na+ | sodium (electrolyte) |
| RAE | right atrial enlargement |
| RCA | right coronary artery |
| RVH | right ventricular hypertrophy |
| SA node | sinus node |

**Clinical Applications:**

| ?allergies | ask for any history of allergy, topical, oral, medication, dyes. |
| ?medical history | taking a full and focused history of the patient's past medical conditions, current illness |
| ?meds | questions medications, prescribed, borrowed, over-the-counter |
| ?vital signs | ask for or assess blood pressure, pulse, respirations, temperature, skin, color temp, and hydration. |
| AAA | abdominal aortic aneurysm |
| ABCs | assessment of airway, breathing, and circulation |
| ALOC | altered level of consciousness |
| ALS | advanced life support |
| AMI | acute myocardial infarction |
| ASAP | as soon as possible |
| ATV | automatic transport ventilator |
| AWMI | anterior wall myocardial infarction |
| BLS | basic life support |
| BP | blood pressure |
| BVM | bag-valve-mask (ventilation device) |
| CC | chief complaint |
| CCU | coronary care unit |
| CHF | congestive heart failure |
| COPD | chronic obstructive pulmonary disease, aka COLD |

| | |
|---|---|
| | (Chronic Lung Disease) |
| CPAP | continuous positive airway pressure |
| CPR | cardiopulmonary resuscitation |
| CV | cardioversion |
| defib | defibrillation |
| Epi | Epinephrine |
| ET | endotracheal intubation |
| H/H | hypotension/hypoperfusion |
| HPI | history of present illness |
| Hx | history |
| IABP | intra aortic balloon pump, aka intra aortic counter pulsation device |
| IM | intramuscular |
| IV | intravenous |
| IVPush | rapid intravenous push (as in injection – immediate—no timed delay) |
| IWMI | inferior wall myocardial infarction |
| LR | lactated Ringer's (IV solution) |
| LOC | level of consciousness |
| LWMI | lateral wall myocardial infraction (left) |
| NS | normal saline |
| NTG | nitroglycerin |
| $O_2$ | oxygen |
| (P) | physician, as in communicate with, contact, call for direction, etc. |
| PE | pulmonary embolus |
| PEA | pulseless electrical activity |
| PEEP | positive end expiratory pressure |
| PMH | past medical history |
| PMI | point of maximum impulse |
| PPV | positive pressure ventilation |
| PRN | pro re nata—(Latin) as the occasion arises; when necessary |
| PTCA | percutaneous transluminal coronary angioplasty |
| RVMI | right ventricular myocardial infarction |
| SL | sublingual |
| SOB | shortness-of-breath |

| SQ | subcutaneous |
| s/s | signs and symptoms |
| sync CV | synchronized cardioversion |
| TAR | traumatic aortic rupture |
| tPA | tissue plasminogen activator |
| USA | unstable angina |

**Pacemaker:**

| FTC | failure to capture |
| FTS | failure to sense |
| TCP | transcutaneous pacing |
| R-R | The interval between two intrinsic ventricular complexes |
| R-V | The interval between the intrinsic QRS to the paced ventricular complex. The pacing interval. |
| V-V | The interval between two ventricular paced complexes. |